The Menopause Sourcebook

THIRD EDITION

Also by Gretchen Henkel

Making the Estrogen Decision (Lowell House, 1992)

Marketing Your Clinical Practice—Ethically, Effectively, Economically, with Dr. Neil Baum (Aspen Publishers, 2000)

The Menopause Sourcebook

THIRD EDITION

GRETCHEN HENKEL

Foreword by
PAUL G. STUMPF, M.D.

Contemporary Books

Chicago   New York   San Francisco   Lisbon   London   Madrid   Mexico City
Milan   New Delhi   San Juan   Seoul   Singapore   Sydney   Toronto

Library of Congress Cataloging-in-Publication Data

Henkel, Gretchen
    The menopause sourcebook / Gretchen Henkel ; foreword by Paul G.
Stumpf.— Rev. 3rd ed.
      p. cm.
    Includes bibliographical references and index.
    ISBN 0-7373-0378-6
    1. Menopause—Popular works. I. Title.
RG186 .H463 2001
618.1'75—dc21
                                    2001028832

Contemporary Books

A Division of The **McGraw·Hill** *Companies*

01 02 03 04 05 06 07 08 09 DOC/DOC 09 08 07 06 05 04 03 02 01

International Standard Book Number: 0-7373-0378-6

This book was set in Galliard by Kate Mueller.
Printed and bound by R.R. Donnelley—Crawfordsville.

Cover design by Cheryl Carrington. Cover photo © Tony Stone Images.
Interior design by Kate Mueller / Electric Dragon Productions.

McGraw-Hill Books are available at special quantity discounts to use as premiums and sales
promotions, or for use in corporate training programs. For more information, please write to the
Director of Special Sales, Professional Publishing, McGraw-Hill, Two Penn Plaza, New York,
NY 10121-2998. Or contact your local bookstore.

This book is printed on acid-free paper.

To Richard and Jesse:
You are my happiness.

CONTENTS

Chapter Five
SEX DURING AND AFTER MENOPAUSE   93

Chapter Six
MENOPAUSE AND BEYOND: SHOULD YOU BE WORRIED?   111

Appendix D
HEIGHT AND WEIGHT TABLE   173

FOREWORD

Menopause is a perfectly natural event in women's lives. But only in the last 25 to 30 years has research provided enough real information to form a basis for scientific dialogue about the menopausal transition. It's hard to believe that even in the 1960s a woman was told that her hot flashes were "all in your head." And their doctors sincerely believed that themselves! It wasn't until the 1970s that researchers demonstrated the physical changes that occur with hot flashes. The old information was wrong, and both doctors and patients may have made bad decisions based on that misinformation.

Like decisions in other situations, decisions in medicine are based on evaluating the benefits and risks, the "pros and cons." It's easy to see that doctors evaluate the benefits and risks when they suggest a medical course of action. And it's also clear that patients evaluate the benefits and risks when they decide whether or not to accept a medical suggestion. What has not been so clear is that these evaluations by doctors and patients may include perceived (not necessarily correct) benefits and risks, as well as real (true) benefits and risks. Surveys show that the "information" doctors and patients use in evaluating the benefits and risks of various approaches to menopause is often not correct.

Now, more than ever, women need to be well-informed and up-to-date on the latest medical information that pertains to their situation. More and more information bombards us every day, and it's harder and harder to keep up. Even worse, not all the information we get is correct. So all of us need to be ever more alert to things that just don't make sense, and willing to seek out sources of reliable information.

During the past five years or so, there has been a phenomenal increase in both medical knowledge and access to it, especially in the area of women's health. Magazines and newspapers devote whole sections to health and fitness on a regular basis, and the latest developments in women's health care are regularly reported on television and radio news programs. And, perhaps most notably, the Internet has given millions of people direct access to scientific reports and medical research that were once limited to professionals only.

With this tremendous increase in the availability of medical information, why are books like this still so important? The answer really lies in the question itself: There is so much information that it is nearly impossible for any one individual to sort through it all and identify what is really valuable. In fact, a knowledgeable guide is arguably more important today than ever before. Anyone who uses the Internet for research quickly learns how much of the results can be useless, inapplicable, or just plain wrong. A guide can help us save time and avoid errors.

For example, one of the biggest changes in menopausal health care in the last few years has been the increased interest in alternative and complementary medicine. Even the established pharmaceutical industry has recognized the public's huge interest in herbal preparations and alternatives to drug therapy. But because this arena is so new to the medical community, much of the information has yet to be analyzed using the tools of Western science. We all need guidance in separating the help from the hype as we learn about this exciting new field of health care.

Another reason a book like this is so valuable is that it can help us ask the right questions. In health care, it is often difficult to find answers for ourselves because we are not entirely comfortable with the technical language in which much of the information is presented. It helps to have a "translator" at our side, at least until we find our way around. Due to managed care and other pressures, doctors and health care providers seem to have less time to explain what their patients read or hear about in the media. When we've done our homework in advance, we can make the best use of the small amount of time we usually get to spend with our professionals and focus on our most important questions.

I have always believed that well-informed patients receive the best health care. The old cliche is true: Knowledge *is* power, in medicine as in the rest of life. By taking control of your menopause (or helping someone you love take control of hers), you can

reach the best possible decisions and aim for the best possible out-
come. I hope you will use this book to help you sort through the
vast amount of medical information out there, so that you can participate fully in the decisions that maximize the quality of your life
during and after the menopausal transition.

PAUL G. STUMPF, M.D.
Clinical Professor of Obstetrics,
Gynecology, and Reproductive Sciences,
Robert Wood Johnson Medical School,
New Brunswick, New Jersey; and Jersey Shore
Medical Center, Neptune, New Jersey

ACKNOWLEDGMENTS

My heartfelt thanks go to my editor, Janice Gallagher, whose curiosity helped form the book's quest and whose support kept me going; to physician Paul Stumpf, M.D., who answered countless questions with equanimity and with women's best health at heart; to Bob Ruckman, who went after and lassoed all the pieces of research I asked him to; to Laura Golden Bellotti, whose ear for language and tone inform the final text; to the women who once again unhesitatingly recounted their personal stories of menopause; and to the other researchers and practitioners who generously took time away from their work to contribute to mine.

INTRODUCTION

My first foray into the subject of menopause and hormone replacement therapy began back in 1991 as part of my research for my first book, *Making the Estrogen Decision*. Although the major landmarks of the menopausal transition remain the same, an incredible explosion of information has changed all the road maps. Typing in the word *menopause* on Medline, the premier database of published medical studies maintained by the National Library of Medicine, recently yielded over 20,000 matches! Ten years ago, there might have been at most 25 book titles about menopause and midlife health issues for women. Now, logging on to Amazon and typing in the word *menopause* can yield up to 500 matches. Reflecting the groundswell for alternatives, the words *holistic, homeopathic, natural, healing,* and *gentle* are more likely to be included in book titles on managing the menopausal transition.

In the ensuing years since I first began this research, one other change has occurred on a personal level. The signs and symptoms that I reported on ten years ago are now happening to me. The transition has begun, and there are days when I'm not so sure I'm happy about this!

Women who are facing menopause often have a feeling of uncertainty. They may fear loss of control or feeling "out of sorts." Having no set expectations makes the anticipation worse. While a minority of women report no symptoms of menopause, the usual course is that a woman will begin feeling changes during the *perimenopause* (*peri*, meaning "around"), which can last from two to five years leading up to menopause. One perimenopausal woman complained to me, "I just want to feel like I did before. I don't feel like my old self. I don't *want* things to change!"

But change they most probably will. There is no predicting your own passage through menopause—it may be long or short, bumpy or smooth. Nor can you foresee the time when you will begin it. Some women may be able to rely on their mother's history as foreshadowing, but it does not always follow that a daughter's menopause mimics her mother's pattern. Your mother may have had a hysterectomy, in which case you have no precedent for the timing of a natural menopause, which usually happens around age 50. Many women have had a surgical menopause, in which the ovaries as well as the uterus are removed, and for them menopause is immediate. Carol, now 55, recalls waking up with intense hot flashes the day after her hysterectomy. An early menopause (younger than age 45) is also not uncommon and may take a woman who's been trying to conceive by surprise. Women who have been amenorrheic (without menstrual periods) because of overexercising or anorexia nervosa may be dealing with the same issue of estrogen depletion that a 50-year-old menopausal woman is. In these latter cases, replacing estrogen becomes more important because of the extended number of years without it. So the issues of women who are going through a natural menopause often align with concerns of those younger women who are already dealing with the consequences of estrogen loss.

Dealing with menopause will be both more hopeful and more frustrating for the current generation of midlife women—the "boomers"—than it was for their mothers. "Hopeful" because we're better equipped to ferret out our own health and medical information and able to speak up and act as our own advocates in health care decision-making. "Frustrating" because definitive answers about the best and most effective therapies for bone, heart, breast, and brain health are still unknown. As Carolyn Kaplan, M.D., a reproductive endocrinologist and associate professor at the Emory University School of Medicine in Atlanta points out, the "information is not there." By this, she means the long-term studies that would show whether estrogen replacement is beneficial to heart and bones, and whether it can cause cancer. These are the big questions that have yet to be answered.

In addition, Dr. Kaplan notes, "Women have conquered contraception and child spacing and most feel that there is greater equality in the workforce. But there is still not enough interest in terms of research dollars being directed toward menopause."

Women at this stage in their lives tend to be take-charge people, juggling jobs, families, and social and volunteer activities. Menopause is something we don't control, and that can be annoying. Who can predict when a hot flash is going to happen? Or when you'll have a bad night plagued by insomnia and feel subfunctional the next day? Or how you'll really feel the first time lovemaking becomes unpleasant because you have no vaginal lubrication? These changes can all be manageable, but that doesn't mean you won't have strong emotions about them.

Whenever and however menopausal changes appear, it can be valuable to have information beforehand, and while you're experiencing menopause. Studies have shown that women who are prepared to take charge of their own health care tend to do best through the menopausal passage. Information can function as your survival kit as you negotiate your way through this very important change in your life.

Becoming well informed is not easy. To whom can we turn for reliable, safe, and personalized health care information? For whatever reason, most women are not getting all the information they need about menopause from their doctors. Research has revealed that only about one-third of women in menopause receive education about the process from their doctors. Incursions of managed care, with its emphasis on cost-containment, almost guarantee that the physician's time is at a premium. Nonetheless, the information that needs to be imparted about menopause is often complex and takes some careful discussion. One of the solutions to the scarcity of a doctor's time versus the patient's need for information has been to provide classes, often conducted by nurse practitioners. As Judith H. LaRosa, Ph.D., former deputy director of the Office of Research on Women's Health at the National Institutes of Health, comments, "The nurse is the one who does the counseling. It's absolutely crucial that you get a nursing perspective, too."

In her practice at the University of California at San Francisco, Mt. Zion Faculty Practice gynecology office, Janis Luft, N.P., M.S., believes all perimenopausal women who come into the office should have the information about the health concerns of menopause and what lifestyle changes they need to confront in order to address those health issues.

"Probably the majority of us will live through our 70s into our 80s," Luft points out. "How *well* we live into our 70s and 80s is the issue. . . . All women need to have a health program as they enter menopause."

To have a health program, you'll probably need to put together a health care team of specialists as well as general practitioners on whom you can rely for guidance and counseling. As you seek such resources, you may find yourself confronting a variety of philosophic and economic issues.

For instance, in addition to getting the most out of our health care dollar, many of us have begun to voice concerns about the remedy most recommended by Western medicine for menopause and the years after: hormone replacement therapy (HRT). Many women view HRT, given most commonly in pill form, as drug treatment. They favor looking to alternative solutions, for the following reasons:

• They're uncomfortable about taking a medication for the rest of their lives.

• They're worried about the possible (though still not conclusively proven) link between HRT and cancer.

• They're unwilling to continue with a medication that's adding side effects and discomfort when it should be relieving their symptoms.

Even mainstream Western medicine, which has scoffed at alternative healing methods, has begun to reconsider its stance. Several large medical institutions, such as Memorial Sloan-Kettering Cancer Center in New York City, now have departments of integrative medicine, in which allopathic physicians, those trained in traditional methods of Western medicine, work to integrate their practices with homeopathic and complementary healing techniques. Some physicians now work in affiliation with acupuncturists; some herbalists have clients who also take hormone therapy. Perhaps most important, growing numbers of physicians recognize that a sound health plan requires participation and cooperation between patient and physician. These are the physicians who trust in their patients' intelligence, good sense, and ability to make the right choices when given full information.

This shift in attitude, I'm convinced, has much to do with pressure from consumers. We as women want to know what will work best for us, and we're seeking information in a variety of places. As I researched and gave presentations for my book *Making the Estrogen Decision*, one theme kept recurring: Women are unsure about taking hormones for the rest of their lives. They want to know: Is it possible to do this the "natural" way? Can hormonal and herbal therapies be combined?

In answer to such questions, I formulated the central mission of *The Menopause Sourcebook*: to provide a compendium of resources, both traditional and alternative, to help you cope with the physical and emotional challenges that often accompany menopause. *The Menopause Sourcebook* puts at your fingertips the information you'll need to handle this life-altering event.

If you've had an early or surgical menopause, and can't or won't take estrogen, this sourcebook belongs to you, too. You may not find all your particulars addressed, but you'll learn how to find the most reliable and recent information, what science does and does not know about this aspect of a woman's physiology, and what sort of issues to take into account in formulating your own health plan. The "Best Resources" section at the end of each chapter offers print and organizational sources of information that can become the core of your health plan. Web site addresses and other Internet resources have also been included.

It is my hope that *The Menopause Sourcebook* will be the beginning of your own personal survival kit for menopause—a place to go for referrals, to learn how to assess and evaluate treatments and remedies, practitioners, and attitudes toward aging. This book will provide you with sources of support and suggestions on how to formulate your own health plan with your physician. Remember that not every bit of information is going to apply to you. You should take from this sourcebook what makes sense and is relevant to you. My purpose is also to stimulate you to ask more of the questions necessary so that the decades following your menopausal transition will be ones of health and renewed purposefulness and activity.

I have observed, as have others working in health education and preventive medicine, that women often benefit from sharing experiences and emotions in a supportive and mutually beneficial way. A "menopause management" class I attended at Kaiser Permanente's Sunset Boulevard facility in Los Angeles is an example of how a group can provide a forum for both emotional support and reliable information. Following a two-hour lecture, each woman in the group was asked to share some personal details about why she had come to the class. Most were hesitant at first. Then, as first one and then another of the women began speaking, the others smiled, laughed, or nodded in agreement and recognition:

> *I was taking estrogen for menopause, and seven months later I had to have a breast biopsy for a suspicious lump. I went off the hormones. Now my hot flashes have started again, but I'm still scared to death to take the hormones. I want to know what I can do.*

> *I don't think I'm in menopause yet, but I notice that I've just been so nervous lately, and fearful. Something is changing, but I'm not sure what.*

> *When I was a girl, my mother really helped me with my first period. She talked to me and prepared me for what was going to happen with my body. But now I find I don't have any preparation for menopause. This is just one more stress in my life!*

> *My doctor suggested that I come to this class. I'm starting to get hot flashes and he is in favor of hormones, but I'm not so sure.*

At the end of the discussion period, most of the women reported that they still had questions and would return for the next class meeting for more information. But they could see that they weren't alone—*everyone* in the room had unresolved issues. They had arrived as strangers, feeling isolated with their symptoms. Now they could see that other women were going through a similar quest. Not all their resolutions would be the same. But it was clear that they had taken the first step in managing their menopause: seeking out information and support.

Let *The Menopause Sourcebook* provide you with a support group in writing, guiding you to the information you need and want.

CHAPTER ONE

Information Gathering

I was treated with an array of tranquilizers, antidepressants,
antianxiety drugs, and psychotherapy. But I wasn't getting any
better. . . . My husband and my family tried hard to understand
and to help. . . . They all supported me, but all were floundering
in confusion, as I was.

> Ruth Jacobowitz, coauthor with Wulf Utian, M.D., of Managing
> Your Menopause, on the confusion she underwent before
> correct diagnosis of menopause

I don't like how I feel. I get the feeling that something is "off
center." I just want to feel like I used to.

> Patricia, 47, now in perimenopause

All women need to have a health program as they enter
menopause.

> Janis Luft, N.P., M.S., Mt. Zion Faculty Practice gynecology office,
> University of California at San Francisco

For women today and those of succeeding generations, menopause need no longer be The Great Unknown. Every year, science
is adding (although some think belatedly so) to our knowledge
about the process and how it affects a woman's body and mind.
And although pre- and perimenopausal women may still look toward the transition with some trepidation ("What is going to happen with me? How will I know when it's started?"), much more
information is available to us than was true for our mothers' generation. Somewhere in the abundance of increased resources we
are bound to find at least some solace in the fact that menopause is
a natural process and that all women experience it.

All this increased attention and research does have a downside: We may have too much information to digest. Women may feel overwhelmed by the input and not want to deal with any of it. *The Menopause Sourcebook* will help you frame your own context for midlife health issues and steer you to the resources to fill in the gaps in your information and support.

Menopause at This Point in History

If you're between the ages of 40 and 50, you're part of the largest group of women ever to go through menopause at one time. By the time the last "baby boomer" goes through menopause (sometime around the year 2014), the ranks of women in our population over the age of 50 will swell to more than 50 million.

Whether you're currently premenopausal, menopausal, or postmenopausal, the current focus on women's health means this is definitely an advantageous time to be going through "the change." As has never before been the case, health professionals and research institutions are finally beginning to turn the spotlight on the distinct concerns of half the world's population.

Spotlight on Women's Health

With the passage of the Women's Health Initiative (WHI) in 1991, the National Institutes of Health (NIH) became even more committed to women's health issues. Various research studies (randomized clinical trials, community intervention studies, and a large surveillance study) connected with the Initiative will eventually include 164,500 postmenopausal participants. The WHI, a 15-year, multimillion-dollar endeavor, will address the most common causes of death, disability, and impaired quality of life in postmenopausal women: cardiovascular disease, cancer, and osteoporosis.

The Initiative was established to address the new awareness that the health status of women differs from that of men. For example, women get heart disease about a decade later than men do, but the progression of the disease is different among women and more apt to be fatal with the first heart attack. The Initiative will investigate the reasons for this and other chronic diseases of aging.

In September 1990, the NIH established an Office of Research on Women's Health, which awards research grants to study health and disease processes in women. That office serves to centralize a focus within the NIH on women's health issues and "to establish a science base that will permit reliable diagnoses, effective treatment, and prevention strategies for women," according to Vivian W. Pinn, M.D., associate director for Research on Women's Health. It is hoped that research will yield some comprehensive preventive strategies for the upcoming aging female population.

On October 1, 1997, administration of the WHI was transferred to the National Heart, Lung, and Blood Institute (NHLBI), where it will be managed as a collaborative effort in cooperation with the National Institute of Arthritis and Musculoskeletal and Skin Diseases (NIAMS), the National Cancer Institute (NCI), and the National Institute on Aging (NIA). For information about the WHI on the Internet, consult the "Best Resources" section at the end of this chapter.

If women today are fortunate to be going through menopause at this point in time, our daughters will most likely benefit even more from the current research atmosphere. That's because the studies begun now will bear results in 5, 10, or 15 years and most likely will give future generations more specific information about women and midlife.

The Physician Credibility Gap

Hormone replacement has been found to arrest bone loss following menopause (thus acting as a preventive against the "brittle bones" disease, osteoporosis) and may reduce the risk of heart attack in some women who take it. Nevertheless, many women have trouble trusting the prescription of a therapy for long-term prevention when they may feel healthy at the moment. The reasons for their reluctance are complex but relate in part to the differing agendas of doctors and patients.

Many physicians urge women to take long-term HRT based on a risk profile for osteoporosis (see "Assessing Osteoporosis Risk," on page 126). However, it is impossible to predict who will develop the disease and who will not—we have no crystal ball. "In fact, even when you're talking about osteoporosis," notes Janine

O'Leary Cobb, M.S., editor of *A Friend Indeed* newsletter, "you can have a woman whose bone density is very, very poor, according to all of the objective tests, but who never fractures a bone. And a woman who is well above normal [may have] bone fractures all over the place. So it makes it very hard for me to insist to people that they must follow what the doctors say when the honest doctors have to admit that they're really fumbling around in the dark a great deal of the time."

O'Leary Cobb might be overstating the position. Physicians would argue that we *do* know a great deal more about menopause than we did 20 years ago, and we're learning more every day. The medical literature on menopause-related topics is huge. We're also living in a time when taboos have been lifted. Menopause is not the "silent passage" it was for our mothers and their mothers. And more physicians today recognize the wisdom of listening to their patients.

Still, the plethora of advice, pro and con, can have the opposite effect of empowerment. A woman can feel directed by "shoulds" and feel stressed by having to make a choice. But despite the conflicts it brings up, information is still power. The important thing is to sift through your resources and find what's useful and pertinent for you—and to remember that nothing is set in stone. It is possible to make one choice, then another, as illustrated in "The Decision Tree" (Figure 1-1).

It may be difficult to get to the point where you ask many questions of your physician and urge him or her to try different approaches. Some physicians are not comfortable with a doctor-patient partnership. But women's health care advocates notice that the dynamic is beginning to change. O'Leary Cobb has seen proof of the establishment's openness to alternatives: She was invited to present a paper at the 1993 International Menopause Society Congress in Stockholm on "Why Women Choose Not to Take Hormones."

"Just being asked to give that presentation was for me an enormous breakthrough—and I don't mean for me personally," she says. "The first International Menopause Society Congress I attended was in 1984 in Orlando, and the doctors couldn't have

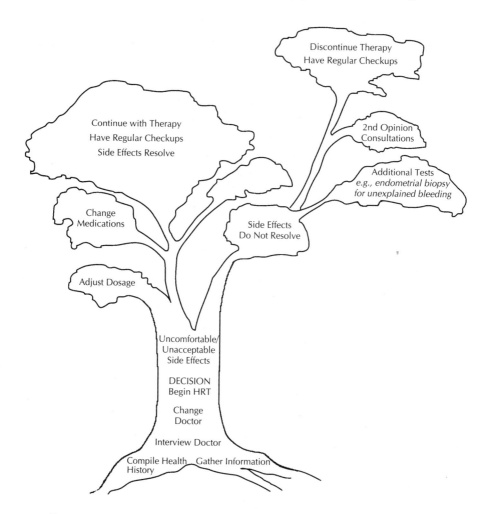

FIGURE 1-1 The Decision Tree *Illustration by Carol Beckerman.*

been less interested in these sorts of [what they would have considered to be] 'marginal issues.'"

Paul Stumpf, M.D., director of the menopause clinic at Jersey Shore Medical Center and a reproductive endocrinologist, concedes that his colleagues have been lacking in how they deal with their menopausal patients. "I think the danger in the past has been that physicians have not provided all of the information that either patients really want but don't know that they want or don't have the context to ask about. Then when patients hear the information somewhere else, or have some difficulty that they weren't warned about, they feel disillusioned about the prescriber who did not provide that information." Another factor, notes Dr. Stumpf, is that the majority of physicians specializing in obstetrics-gynecology (ob/gyn) in this country are male and may have some difficulty in "understanding how significant some of these side effects [of HRT] are. . . . There's a gap in the ability to understand what the patient is really concerned about. I think the way that that's going to solve itself is that almost 60 percent of ob/gyn residents are now women, so in 10 or 20 years, that whole profile will change. I guess what I would always advise is: Anytime you feel the doc's not listening to you, that's the time to go ask somebody else."

You are the best judge of how you're treated in the doctor's office. Despite Dr. Stumpf's assessment of women changing the face of the profession, a gynecologist's gender does not automatically convey a certain type of treatment. Men can be compassionate; women can be impatient. The point is to find someone (or several someones) with whom you feel comfortable. In Chapter 3, you'll learn more about putting your health care team together.

Must I Deal with Menopause?

Many women would prefer not to think about menopause ahead of time. ("Menopause? I'll worry about it when I get there," says a 40-something office manager.) Of course, menopause itself is not life-threatening. For some women, it's a minor blip on the screen of life. But for others, the signs and symptoms of menopause can deliver a sudden and rude wake-up call. Because of the changes set in motion during menopause, there are good reasons to prepare ahead of time to deal with its consequences.

The first step is to learn about the process of menopause. Chapter 3 explains the variety of menopausal signs and symptoms. But for now, a brief description: Menopause doesn't happen in one single moment, month, or year. Rather, it takes place over a period of years. From our 30s onward, our bodies are continually undergoing changes leading up to menopause. Our egg supply gradually diminishes. As we move into our 40s, ovulation, the main source of estrogen production, becomes erratic. Periods may come closer together or further apart, produce light or heavy bleeding, or sometimes a flooding with no warning. (Some gynecologists now believe that changes in premenstrual syndrome [PMS] in the 40s actually signal that a woman is in perimenopause—the two to five years before cessation of menstruation.) Finally, when a woman is without a period for a year, she is postmenopausal. It is then that her body's landscape changes.

Some of the changes associated with menopause are more visible than others. Drying skin and decreased vaginal lubrication are pretty noticeable, while the condition of your bones, heart, and blood vessels is not as readily apparent. In fact, menopause produces changes in almost all of your body's major systems, and they won't go away by your ignoring them. As with any major life change, you bring to this juncture a lifetime of physical health history, attitudes about your body and health, and coping styles. If you take advantage of the information available and plan ahead, you can reduce your uncertainties and help yourself enjoy a better transition.

By the time you hit the age of menopause, your body has already shown signs of aging: Weight has become harder to lose, and fat redistributes around your middle; your skin has lost some of its elasticity and has begun to wrinkle more; you may require reading glasses or bifocals. All of these changes are natural. While we may resist them, they are going to happen anyway. It's how we adapt to the menopausal transition that makes a difference in how our bodies undergo these changes.

This book is designed to help you assess your menopausal health and formulate your own health plan. The steps are:

- Evaluate your current health status. (See Chapter 2, "Entering Menopause: Where Do You Stand?")

- Understand what menopause means. (See Chapter 3, "Is This It? The Signs and Symptoms of Menopause.")

- Form a plan or strategy for dealing with menopausal symptoms. (See Chapter 4, "The Physical Effects of Menopause: Managing Your Symptoms.")

- Deal with your shifting sexuality. (See Chapter 5, "Sex During and After Menopause.")
- Evaluate what the depletion of estrogen might mean for your long-term health. (See Chapter 6, "Menopause and Beyond: Should You Be Worried?")
- Understand and deal with potential psychological stress during menopause. (See Chapter 7, "The Body/Mind Connection: Menopause and Emotional Stress.")
- Consider your place in the world as you age. (See Chapter 8, "Integrating Change and Exploring Opportunity.")
- Throughout all these stages and chapters, evaluate what you can *realistically* change—and what you can't.

Think Exception, Not the Rule

What can a woman expect when she goes through menopause? There are a number of general signs and symptoms and one definitive one—the end of menstruation for one year, which is the clinical definition of menopause. But as with all generalizations, rigid adherence to a profile of symptoms will not be helpful when talking about each individual woman. Remember that menopause, or *cessation of menses,* is part of a reproductive continuum that began before you were born. In Chapter 3, you'll learn about the processes that trigger menopause.

For now, keep in mind that the average age of menopause is 50. For a minority of menopausal women (researchers have put the number between 5 and 10 percent), the transition will be asymptomatic, with no overt signs or symptoms. Margie, a very energetic entrepreneur and now 67, recalls, "I think I had one or two hot flashes. I was about 51, and I remember thinking, 'Oh, so that's what it is.' But then I didn't have any more. That was it!" Despite her minimal hot flashes, Margie's body was making internal adjustments to the depletion of estrogen, and at the age of 59 she began using a transdermal estrogen patch to guard against bone loss.

Most women (70 to 85 percent) will experience hot flashes and vaginal dryness, and a large minority will have night sweats. The potential for variety is great during menopause, because each woman's physical makeup, family health history, and cultural environment are distinct.

You may have had one or several children, or no children at all. You may have enjoyed relatively good health throughout your reproductive years, with normal Pap smears, normal pregnancies, and no abnormal bleeding. Or you may have been plagued with bleeding fibroids and the threat of hysterectomy at a young age. You may have required hormonal replacement to counter amenorrhea. These are the kinds of details from your individual health history that must be taken into account when you begin to formulate your health plan. When it comes to menopause, every woman is unique.

Your Health Care Attitudes

You may be very well informed about menopause, or you may be getting most of your information from anecdotes related by friends. Wherever you are in the continuum, more information will probably help.

What about your doctor? Do you trust him or her? Have you achieved a working partnership? Menopause is a time when you may need to rely on your physician's skills even more. With the amount of data accumulating in the scientific literature on menopause, it is an advantage to have a physician who can help you interpret what various studies mean in your particular case.

When they start learning about the pros and cons of HRT, many women feel frustrated. They want to know how doctors can ask them to "hang in there" with uncomfortable side effects when the results can't be guaranteed. Some women feel they aren't getting enough information about alternative treatments from their doctors and have sought help elsewhere. Part of your own information gathering about menopause may include looking at nonhormonal therapies and treatments.

The Eastern and Alternative Ways

Among women I interviewed, a sizable percentage voiced disillusionment with what Western medicine is offering them. Countless women use herbs, acupuncture, biofeedback, homeopathic remedies, and other treatments to get them through the menopausal transition. While it's tempting to assume that all so-called natural and alternative treatments are at most curative and at the very least harmless, that is not always the case. I would urge women to investigate an herbal practitioner as carefully as they would a new gynecologist. This is not easy, of course, because accreditation is not as standardized within the alternative healing community. Women should approach any treatment with what Janine O'Leary Cobb calls "a healthy skepticism." You should beware, for instance, of a practitioner who totally negates Western medicine, or whose offices are not spotlessly clean, or who claims to be the path to perfect health. Reputable naturopaths like Los Angeles acupuncturist Janet Zand will tell you that achieving "perfect health" is impossible. "Life is ever-changing," she notes. "[Promising perfect health] is promising to be able to control that person's life. . . . How you feel when you're premenopausal, how you feel when you're perimenopausal, and how you feel when you are postmenopausal—you're going to have different requirements during all of those phases."

Working in consumer education and health fraud, John H. Renner, M.D., was a family practice physician and clinical professor of medicine at the University of Missouri in Kansas City and investigated practitioners who take advantage of patients who may be disillusioned with traditional Western medicine. Many in the "alternative" field are actually no more than good salespeople, Dr. Renner believed. "People have a double standard of levels of evidence or proof, requiring almost no proof from these super salespeople and demanding absolute perfection and guarantee and truth from the scientific community. That just isn't logical." As a general guide for evaluating a therapy, Dr. Renner advised consumers to look at proposed therapies as described in Table 1-1.

Dr. Renner urged consumers to use caution when trying various alternative remedies. "Many people," he said, "are taking all kinds of things at the same time. I think some people think they are 'super healthy' if they are taking 50 pills a day." This was not unusual in his experience. Any substance taken orally goes through your intestinal tract, is processed by the liver, and enters your bloodstream. The label of "natural" is not a guarantee that a product is harmless. Many natural herbal products are imported from other countries where no food and drug regulations exist. Once they arrive here, a "nutritional supplement" is not counted as a drug product and is not regulated by the Food and Drug Administration (FDA).

In general, Western medicine has not been accepting of natural remedies, most of which fall into Dr. Renner's "unproven" category. Alan R. Gaby, M.D., in his book *Preventing and Reversing Osteoporosis,* offers an explanation for this. Studies of non-patented substances are not in the scientific literature, he states, because "most research grant money comes from the pharmaceutical industry and from other organizations that have a vested interest in studying patentable substances or in promoting a particular point of view."

Dr. Stumpf has noticed an increasing cynicism among patients toward the medical community. "I'm not sure what the wellspring of that cynicism is," he says, "but I have to feel that somewhere at the bottom of it all is that we haven't communicated well enough for patients to trust us at that level. Certainly all of us have the

Table 1-1   Classifications of Remedies and Therapies

Type of Therapy	Most Notable Characteristics
Folklore	Home remedies handed down from generation to generation; generally safe, but have not been submitted to scientific scrutiny.
Quackery	Best known for its testimonials—positive and negative; characterized by oversimplification and its ability to market products.
Unproven	Remedies that may work but that have not been investigated.
Investigational	Characterized by peer review, good record keeping, criticism of data at the scientific level.
Proven	Effectiveness has been proven by scientific peers; is now ready for general public consumption; debates and examination still take place; may be proven false at a later date.

experience with individual patients of establishing a good level of communication where we're willing to challenge their belief system and they're willing to bring new information to us. But globally, I wonder what we're doing wrong as a profession that leads to such an inability to find reasons to trust us. When I respond that I don't have information about a certain alternative remedy, patients sometimes respond with, 'Oh, you doctors are so close-minded, trying to protect your own territory.' Hormone replacement therapy has about 45 years' worth of medical literature, good and bad, and because of what patients perceive to be the unknown elements, they will go to the local health food store, take something off the shelf that has virtually no quality control, and pay good money for that. It's an amazing set of belief patterns."

The lack of data on complementary and alternative medicine is slowly beginning to change. The Office of Alternative Medicine, newly renamed the National Center for Complementary and Alternative Medicine (NCCAM), has an increased budget for funding studies on herbal products and healing remedies. After much controversy, the NIH has determined that it is possible to use standard scientific testing (comparing the effects of a new compound to those of a placebo) to assess complementary treatments.

Alternative practitioners often promote taking plant estrogens (phytoestrogens) instead of synthetic or manufactured estrogens as a protection against osteoporosis. According to Dr. Renner, osteoporosis "is a perfect illness to 'scam' somebody because it takes such a long time to evaluate. Phytoestrogens are common in nature. Even garlic and alfalfa have some estrogen. But the *dosage* is what counts, and the only dosages that we know how to measure are the ones that have been evaluated in clinical studies."

Until we have reliable research data about herbal products, it's probably a good idea to proceed cautiously in this area. In Chapter 4, you'll get some idea of the best way to use certain herbal teas and products. What course you take, what remedies you seek, is ultimately up to you. In this book, you will find ways to assess how a particular treatment or strategy fits with your lifestyle and health risk assessments.

You Are Not Alone

What happened to me should not happen to any woman, anywhere.

Ruth Jacobowitz, writing in the introduction of Managing Your Menopause, *about her ordeals with menopause*

Ruth Jacobowitz started menopause in 1985, when the subject was not widely covered in the media. She found herself floundering for a time, not knowing what was happening to her and suspecting that perhaps she might be "going crazy." The resources for menopausal women are expanding daily—books (more than 500 titles now in print), magazine articles, seminars, support groups, and especially Internet resources abound. Some of these resources are reliable, some are not.

Researchers have noted an explosion of consumers consulting Internet sources for their health and medical information. According to one market research firm, Cyber Dialogue, Inc., more than 22 million Americans used their computers to seek medical information in 1998, a number expected to increase by about 70 percent a year into the foreseeable future. Not every site contains scientifically validated information, according to one orthopedic oncologist who did a test survey of the Internet using the name of a common pediatric bone cancer, Ewing's sarcoma. Dr. J. Sybil Biermann of the University of Michigan's Medical School found that one-third of the sites visited had no reference to peer review, considered a hallmark of reliable information, and 6 percent of those sites had information that was totally incorrect. For more information on obtaining reliable health information, consult the "Best Resources" section at the end of Chapter 4.

Whether your menopause is at hand or five years off, your best insurance for a healthy and fruitful transition is to begin gathering your materials now. In Chapter 2, you'll start with a premenopause checkup. Before you do, you might want to check out the following "Best Resources" list to help give you an overview.

Best Resources

In this section, I have listed some titles to help you in your information-gathering stage. These are good all-round reference books on menopause. The newsletters provide a way to stay current with new research, and their "Letters to the Editors" sections present other voices of women at this stage of life. It may be helpful to read such stories as you near your own menopause.

Books

Dr. Susan Love's Hormone Book: Making Informed Choices About Menopause, by Susan M. Love, M.D., and Karen Lindsey. Times Books (Random House), New York, 1998; paperback, 375 pages; $15.00.

Written in the same direct, no-nonsense style as her *Breast Book,* this book by Dr. Love covers a wealth of both mainstream and alternative remedies for all the changes of menopause.

Managing Your Menopause, by Wulf H. Utian, M.D., Ph.D., and Ruth S. Jacobowitz. A Fireside Book (Simon and Schuster), New York, 1990; paperback, 214 pages; $10.00.

Written by the founder of the North American Menopause Society and his coauthor, this book introduces the physiology of menopause and details the elements of the Utian Menopause Management Program. Although some criticize the emphasis on diet and nutrition and "total body care," as opposed to more on menopause itself, the book offers much helpful information and is a good overview for women in midlife.

Menopause and Midlife Health, by Morris Notelovitz, M.D., Ph.D., and Diana Tonnessen. St. Martin's Press, New York, 1994; paperback, 494 pages; $16.95.

A comprehensive reference for all aspects of women's midlife health, from contraception to hormone replacement, to figuring your ratio of body fat to total body weight. Contains voluminous charts, questionnaires, and programs to start exercise, alcohol and smoking reduction, and so on. Weight and height tables are more inclusive than the 1983 Metropolitan Insurance tables. Written by a top researcher in the field.

Menopause: A Guide for Women and Those Who Love Them, by Winnifred B. Cutler, Ph.D., and Celso-Ramon Garcia, M.D. W. W. Norton & Co., New York, 1993 (revised edition); paperback, 431 pages; $14.95.

A comprehensive look at menopause and other midlife health issues. The tone is perhaps more scientifically oriented than the previous two books mentioned, but it is thorough, reasoned, and well researched. A good addition to your menopause library.

Menopause: A Positive Approach, by Rosetta Reitz. Penguin Books, New York, 1979; paperback reprint, 265 pages; $11.95.

This is one of the original books about menopause written from a woman's point of view. An author and blues historian, Reitz includes factual material about menopause interwoven with her own and other women's stories. Successfully combines self-help items such as a menopausal symptoms diary with a historical examination of the politics of menopause and aging.

Newsletters

A Friend Indeed Publications, Inc.
P.O. Box 260
Pembina, ND 58271-0260
8 issues a year/$30.00 [$40.00 outside the U.S.]
(204) 989-8028 phone
(204) 989-8029 fax
www.afriendindeed.ca

Founder and former editor Janine O'Leary Cobb now acts as an editorial consultant for the newsletter she began 16 years ago. The current editor is Sari Tudiver, Ph.D. Each issue features a full-length article on one aspect of menopause and midlife health (a recent back issue on progestins and progesterone is available on their Web site), as well as regular columns. This is a reasoned, intelligent publication, with a tone that lets you know you're among friends who care. The editors approach topics with a healthy skepticism about mainstream medical recommendations, but do not herald herbal and alternative treatments as ultimate panaceas either. Especially wonderful are the letters from readers that appear in a regular section called "The Exchange." Here you'll read about readers' myriad menopausal symptoms, as well as how women have come to grips with them. Summaries of recent relevant journal studies appear regularly in the "Hot Flashes" column.

Harvard Women's Health Watch
Monthly/$32.00 per year
P.O. Box 420235
Palm Coast, FL 32142
(800) 829-5921

Health After 50
(Published by Johns Hopkins University)
Monthly/$28.00 per year
P.O. Box 420179
Palm Coast, FL 32142
(800) 829-0422

Internet Resources

You can do a search using the keyword *menopause* (via Yahoo!, Alta Vista, dogpile.com, or other search engines) and find a wealth of listings. Here are a few with good, verifiable content:

1. Doctor's Guide to Menopause Information and Resources
   Provides the latest medical news and information for "patients and/or friends of patients diagnosed with menopause." Discussion groups, medical alerts, and other categories are also useful.
   www.pslgroup.com/menopause.htm
2. OBGYN.net
   A physician-reviewed service for medical professionals, industry representatives, and perimenopausal and menopausal women.
   www.obgyn.net
3. iVillage.com
   This online magazine for women, chock-full of interesting features and resources, contains a category called "Better Health," which contains physician-reviewed consumer articles

on all aspects of health, including midlife and menopause.
www.ivillage.com

4. Home page of the Women's Health Initiative
   Background information, an overview of the WHI's objectives
   and mission statement, as well as links to Medline, the National Library of Medicine's database, and current information
   on participating in clinical trials and observational studies are
   some of the resources available at this Web site.
   www.nhlbi.nih.gov/index.htm

CHAPTER TWO

Entering Menopause: Where Do You Stand?

The 40s are the best yet, aren't they? I've never been happier with my work or with my family.
Nancy, 42, owner of a public relations firm

I watched my mother go through hell with menopause. I'm just dreading it and wondering: Is that what I'm in for, too?
Kathleen, 43

I don't even want to bring up the subject of menopause with my doctor. I know he's "into hormones" and I'm just afraid it'll give me breast cancer.
Beth, 47 and perimenopausal

If you're 40-something, you've heard the news by now: Menopause is on its way. And it's happening in big numbers. The U.S. Census Bureau's 1990 figures put the number of women presently in the 50 to 59 age group at 11 million. By the year 2010, that number will triple when the 20 million women who are part of what Dr. Judith Reichman calls "the menopause boomers" join the ranks of the over-50 population. To give those figures even more immediacy, the North American Menopause Society estimates that four thousand women become menopausal every day in North America.

You probably don't need the media reminding you, though. Like Linda, 44, whose PMS in the last three years has intensified, creating disruption and havoc in her life, you may be all too aware that your body is already changing.

During the several years leading up to menopause and the years of transition, often referred to as perimenopause, your body is readying itself for the switch to a nonreproductive stage. This can be a time when premenstrual and menstrual symptoms— mood swings, bloating, pain with menstruation—become exacerbated and cause great distress. Many women experience a shortening of their menstrual cycles. That's because the follicular phase, when an egg is being prepared to be released by the ovary, is shortened. This phase of shortened menstrual cycles moves later into a transitional menstrual pattern characterized by longer intervals between shorter cycles. In Chapter 3, the hallmarks of menopause will be discussed more fully. In this chapter, we'll focus on which health factors a woman should be monitoring as she goes through her 40s and perimenopause.

Now is a good time to think about the kinds of health issues that could affect your menopausal transition. As you'll learn in Chapter 4, the decline of estrogen production has long-term consequences for many of your body's systems—circulatory, skeletal, reproductive. This is the reason that many physicians believe women should go on long-term hormone replacement therapy: to ensure quality of life for the quarter century or so that they can expect to live beyond menopause.

Whether or not you take hormones will be your individual decision. It is possible to have a positive impact on both your present and future health, however, by doing a personal health assessment now. This chapter is designed to help you get a clearer picture of your general health and decide what changes you can make to become even healthier. Having knowledge about your body is a great way to empower yourself and to make your transition as smooth as possible. Information that you acquire now could also help allay any anxieties you might have about this potentially unsettling phase of your middle years.

By the time you've reached 40, you've probably had several thorough physical examinations. But some women, who enjoy remarkably trouble-free health, may visit their doctors infrequently, perhaps seeing their gynecologists only for their yearly Pap smear.

In this chapter, you'll get an idea of additional screening tests that would be good for you at this time of your life and of some preventive measures you can begin to take now to make the menopausal transition smoother and the years beyond healthier.

When it comes to the major diseases affecting midlife and older women (heart disease, osteoporosis, cancer), early detection is the key to long-term survival and quality of life. Getting a baseline mammogram, for example, is a good idea after age 40. But many women I know put it off. The reason? Fear. Unfortunately, fear can keep you from taking life-saving actions. The "Heart Test for Women," which begins on page 27, is another example of how to use early detection to advantage.

The 40s appear to be a particularly opportune time for self-assessment and lifestyle adjustments. In the May 1993 cover article for *The Atlantic*, writer Winifred Gallagher interviewed psychologists and sociologists at length about the verity of many commonly held beliefs about midlife. The consensus of Gallagher and the experts she interviewed was that these notions—that a midlife crisis is unavoidable, that sex fades after 40, that many people suffer from fears of aging—are myths. In fact, many of the experts interviewed have found that the 40s in particular are a decade of increased productivity and confidence for most people. Both men and women appear to reach a stage of mastery in their careers and on the whole tend to be more realistic about comparing themselves to others, setting their own goals independent of outside standards, and attaining success and satisfaction in life.

This rosy report doesn't mean you're weird if you are afraid of aging. Most people would admit they don't like to think about diminished energies and limited capacity; many would prefer to get fewer wrinkles and sags. Physical aging can often trigger a reassessment of priorities. Then, too, midlife can be a time when additional pressures are heaped on your plate. Sally, 42, has watched her mother become more dependent on her since her father's death. "Now I hear about the daily complaints," she notes. "And it's hard—I've got my kids, my husband, my work, and now I'm her confidante, too."

But pressures don't have to get to the boiling point. According to Ann Kearney-Cooke, an adjunct professor of psychology at the University of Cincinnati and a psychologist in private practice, "One thing that I observe about working with women at middle age—that I don't find as much with younger women—is that they're wiser, they're smarter. They tend to have experience under their belts and they work really well."

Paul Stumpf, M.D., of Jersey Shore Medical Center, has noticed that women "are much more conscious of menopause itself and come to us earlier, before their periods have stopped and they're miserable with hot flashes, to ask about what to anticipate. I think there's more of an awareness of the fact that menopause is not a single moment in time, a doorway that you walk through and then it's done—but more of an understanding that there is this whole variable period of time in the transition."

With those endorsements in mind, let's begin our personal health self-assessment. Here we'll be concerned with the state of your bones, your heart and cardiovascular system, and your self-image. Remember to take only the advice that seems to apply to you. Many of us are already dealing with existing health problems. It's important not to "grade" yourself or allow this health information to become yet another thing that you fear you're not handling quite "right."

Bones, Calcium, and Exercise: Do You Have the Right Prescription?

Your bones are living tissue: Old bone cells are constantly being broken down and replaced with new bone cells in a process called *bone remodeling*. Most bone mass is built during childhood and adolescence. Unless you've had a condition that depletes the bone mass, your bones continue to increase slightly in density until the age of 35. At that time, both men and women begin to lose a little—up to 1 percent a year—of their bone density. Men usually start with greater bone mass, however, so if they get osteoporosis (about 10 percent of the total cases are men), it usually occurs much later in life.

Scientists have discovered that estrogen is crucial to the bone remodeling process, aiding the body's absorption of calcium to contribute to bone mineral content. When estrogen levels fall after menopause, the delicate balance of bone remodeling is tipped toward the side of *resorption,* or breaking down of bone. Women need to be especially careful to supply their bones with enough calcium and vitamin D both before and after menopause. It's also wise to include green leafy vegetables, whole grains, and beans in your diet. Those foods contain substantial amounts of magnesium, a crucial mineral for calcium absorption. If you don't absorb the calcium you ingest, kidney stones or calcium deposits may form in your arteries and joints. (See Appendix A, "Calcium-Rich Foods," and Appendix B, "Comparison of Calcium Supplements.")

As you move through your 40s toward menopause, keep in mind also that your digestive tract is changing. Foods are absorbed and processed in different ways. You can become lactose-intolerant, which means that your body cannot tolerate the sugars in milk. Many commercial products are now available, from milk to cottage cheese to hard cheeses, made for people with this problem. Or you may want to cut dairy products from your diet and replace them with calcium supplements.

The best time to build strong bones is during childhood and adolescence, so if you've got young children and teenagers, urge them to continue drinking milk. But you can take steps at any stage of adult life to increase your chances of preventing osteoporosis.

A few lifestyle changes now could save you from losing too much bone after menopause and becoming a candidate for the bone-thinning and stress fractures of this disease, which can go undetected until it's too late. In Chapter 6, you'll learn why doctors and public health experts are so concerned about osteoporosis.

In addition to your estrogen status, the three key elements for keeping bones healthy and strong, according to the National Osteoporosis Foundation, are:

1. Eating a balanced diet rich in calcium, 1,000 mg (milligrams) a day for premenopausal women; up to 1,500 mg after menopause if not taking hormone replacement (see Appendix A for a list of calcium-rich foods).

2. Engaging in weight-bearing exercise two to three times a week, for at least 20 minutes at a time. These activities include walking, jogging, dancing, aerobics, and racquet sports.

3. Changing any adverse lifestyle habits that can affect your bone health. The habits most deleterious to your bones are smoking cigarettes (which is unhealthful for many additional reasons) and drinking alcohol. Both smoking and alcohol can actually deplete the calcium in your system, and your body will then extract calcium from your bones. Many experts also add caffeine to the list, because it, too, can increase the amount of calcium excreted in the urine (an indication it's not being absorbed into your system).

If you don't know how to begin assessing your bone health, start by talking with your doctor about osteoporosis. Do you have special risk factors that mean you've already lost a dangerous percentage of bone mass? Among those in this high-risk group are people who have taken steroids for extended periods of time (asthmatics and transplant patients, for example), women who have been amenorrheic, those with eating disorders such as bulimia or anorexia nervosa, those who have had an early surgical menopause (oophorectomy—removal of the ovaries) and who have not taken estrogen, and women with a sedentary lifestyle.

As a woman in midlife, ask the questions in the box on page 25 when you see your doctor for your annual checkup.

In the meantime, maintaining a moderate level of physical exertion may help to keep your bones dense. Doing weight-bearing exercise puts stress on your bones, stimulating the buildup of bone tissue. Remember to support your physical activity program with adequate rest, nutrition, and calcium intake.

Heart, Blood Vessels, and Estrogen

If you're not a smoker, don't have diabetes, aren't obese, and don't have hypertension, being a premenopausal woman is good temporary insurance against heart disease. That women have fewer heart attacks and less heart disease before the age of 50 than do men has tended to cloud the issue of heart disease, however. As women go through menopause and lose estrogen's protective effects on their circulatory systems, they quickly take on the risk factors for cardiovascular disease that have traditionally been perceived as belonging mostly to men.

In fact, cardiovascular disease (heart attacks and vascular events like stroke) is the number one cause of death for women over the age of 50. Every year, approximately 500,000 women die from heart attacks and strokes, compared with 260,000 deaths of women from all types of cancer.

According to Carolyn L. Murdaugh, Ph.D., R.N., acting scientific director, National Institute of Nursing Research, and chief of the Laboratory for the Study of Human Responses to Health and Illness at the National Institutes of Health, heart disease is fatal more often in women than in men. She attributes this to the fact that women are older when they develop coronary artery

---

Questions You Should Ask Your Doctor

- Should I worry about preventing osteoporosis?

- How can I strengthen or preserve my bones?

- What type of exercise is best?

- How much calcium do I need, and what are the best sources of calcium?

- How can I help my family members learn about osteoporosis?

- Should I have a bone mass measurement?

- How often should I have my bone mass measured?

- Do I need to consider medical treatment? If yes, what are the benefits and risks of these treatments?

- When should I come in for a follow-up exam?

Source: "Talking with Your Doctor About Osteoporosis," © 1992, National Osteoporosis Foundation.

disease, are referred to treatment later, and are admitted and transferred to hospitals later than men are. Unfortunately, physicians often pursue less aggressive treatment and fewer invasive procedures with female patients who have heart disease symptoms than with their male counterparts.

Kathy, now 49, is a case in point. At the age of 44, she went to her local hospital's emergency room with chest pains. The doctor on duty told her she was "too young" for heart disease and didn't even do an electrocardiogram (EKG). Kathy insisted that something was wrong. Two years later she underwent bypass surgery.

Edward B. Diethrich, M.D., medical director of the Arizona Heart Institute, is one of the growing numbers of researchers who speak frequently about the dangers of ignoring the signs of heart disease in women. "One of the things that must occur in the educational process for women is to broadcast the fact that they don't have this for-lifetime protection that fortunately most of them have before menopause," he says. "Women need to understand that they *do* get this disease. And while it may have different presentations and different manifestations than for males, when they get it [about 10 years later than males], the prognosis is worse. The interventions, when they are done, are going to be less satisfactory than in the male, and recovery is typically longer, too." Women need to educate themselves about the signs of early heart disease, and their doctors might be well advised to do the same. If you're in good health, Dr. Diethrich advises getting your cholesterol levels checked once a year.

The medical profession now realizes that heart disease in women must be taken more seriously. Symposia such as the one held in the fall of 1993 by the Los Angeles Chapter of the American Heart Association on heart disease in women, minorities, and children help to educate physicians, nurses, and the media.

It's also up to us as sensible health care consumers to take heart disease seriously. Perhaps you've never given heart disease a second thought. You may have kept your weight down and modified your diet to lower the fat content of your meals. But do you know about the other factors that could have an effect on your heart health after menopause? The following "Heart Test for Women" was developed at the Arizona Heart Institute and Foundation to educate women about their risk factors. To find out your risk level, take the test by adding the numbers that apply to your situation, totaling all the categories, and then consulting the scoring ranges at the end:

∾   ∾   ∾

HEART TEST FOR WOMEN

Category	Score
Age	
51 and over	5
35 to 50	2
34 and under	0
Family History	
Have any of your parents, brothers, or sisters had a heart attack, stroke, or heart bypass surgery at:	
Age 55 or before	5
Age 56 or after	3
None or don't know	0
Personal History	
Have you had:	
A heart attack	20
Angina, heart bypass surgery, angioplasty, stroke, or blood vessel surgery	10
None of the above	0
Smoking	
Current smoker: How many cigarettes per day?	
5 or more	20
4 or fewer	10
If you are a smoker currently taking oral contraceptives and are:	
Under 35	2
35 and over	5

If you are an ex-smoker who quit less than 2 years ago, how many cigarettes per day did you smoke?

5 or more	10
4 or fewer	5

If you have never smoked or quit more than 2 years ago   0

Blood Pressure

If you have had your blood pressure taken in the last year, was it:

Elevated or high (either or both readings above160/95 mmHg)	6
Borderline (between 140/90 and 160/95 mmHg)	3
Normal (below 140/90 mmHg) or don't know	0

Hormone Status

If you have undergone natural menopause, your age at its start:

41 or older	1
40 or younger	2

If you have had a total hysterectomy, your age when it was done:

41 or older	1
40 or younger	3
If you take an oral estrogen supplement	subtract 2
If you are still menstruating	subtract 1

Exercise

Do you engage in any aerobic activity, such as brisk walking, jogging, bicycling, or swimming, for more than 20 minutes?

Less than once a week	6
1 or 2 times a week	3
3 or more times a week	0

Blood Fats

If you have had your cholesterol and blood fat levels checked in the last year, score your risk here:

Over 240 mg/dl	6
200 to 240 mg/dl	3
Cholesterol under 200 mg/dl	0

If your HDLs (high-density lipoproteins) are lower than 45   1

Or, if you know your cholesterol-to-HDL ratio, use this section to score your risk:

7.1 and above	6
3.6–7.0	3
3.5 or below	0

If you do not know your cholesterol and blood fat levels, use this section to score your risk. Which of the following best describes your eating pattern? (Use score from only one section.):

High fat: red meat, fast foods, and/or fried foods daily; more than 7 eggs per week; regular consumption of butter, whole milk, and cheese   6

Moderate fat: red meat, fast foods, and/or fried foods 4 to 6 times per week; 4 to 7 eggs weekly; regular use of margarine, vegetable oils, and/or low-fat dairy products   3

Low fat: poultry, fish, and little or no red meat, fast foods, fried foods, or saturated fats; fewer than 3 eggs per week; minimal margarine and vegetable oils; primarily nonfat dairy products   0

Diabetes

If you have diabetes (blood sugar level above 140 mg/dl), your age when you found out:

40 or before	6
41 or older	4
Do not have diabetes	0

Body Mass

Calculate your body mass index with the following formula:

Weight (pounds): _____ × 0.45 = _____ (W)
Height (inches): _____ × 0.025 = _____ (H)

Divide (W) by the square of (H) or
$W \div H \times H$ = Body Mass Index (BMI).

W _____ ÷ (H × H) _____ = _____ (BMI)

Example: A woman weighs 120 pounds and is 5 feet 6 inches (66 inches) tall:

$120 \times 0.45 = 54$ (W) $66 \times 0.025 = 1.65$ (H)

$W \div H \times H = 54 \div 1.65 \times 1.65 = 54 \div 2.72 = 19.8$ BMI.

If your BMI is 27 or greater	2
If your BMI is below 27	0

Now measure your waist and hips and divide your waist measurement by your hip girth to calculate your hip-to-waist ratio:

(waist) _____ ÷ (hips) _____ = _____

Example: Your waist is 26 and your hips are 36: $26 \div 36 = 0.7$.

If your waist-to-hip ratio is 0.8 or greater	1
If your ratio is 0.79 or less	0

Stress

Are you easily angered and frustrated:

Most of the time	6
Some of the time	3
Rarely	0

TOTAL SCORE _____

What Your Risk Factor Score Means

15 points or below: Low Risk
Congratulations! Maintain your heart-healthy status by watching your weight, blood pressure, and blood fat (cholesterol and HDL) levels; get regular checkups and don't smoke. Retake this test every year to monitor your heart-health risk profile.

16 to 32 points: Medium Risk
Our experience indicates that your medium risk level warrants attention. Personal factors or lifestyle habits may be increasing your vulnerability to heart disease. We strongly recommend you schedule an appointment with your doctor for an evaluation, and take this test with you to get advice on how you can improve your heart-health status.

33 points or above: High Risk
Your potential for experiencing a heart attack or stroke is significant. You must take action NOW. If you are not already being treated for heart disease, we urgently advise that you see your doctor immediately and take this test with you. You must seek ways to reduce your risk!

Source: "Heart Test for Women," © 1992; Arizona Heart Institute and Foundation, Phoenix, Arizona. Reprinted by permission.

❧   ❧   ❧

Don't Forget Breast Health

Of the women diagnosed with new cases of breast cancer each year, the majority, or 77 percent, are over the age of 50. Women between the ages of 20 and 29 account for only 0.3 percent of breast cancer cases. The American Cancer Society estimates that for 1999 175,000 new cases of invasive breast cancer were diagnosed. Alarming breast cancer statistics affect the anxiety level of every American woman. Knowing your risk factors and making sure you get the proper screening can go a long way toward easing your mind. Because we still do not know how to prevent breast cancer, early detection is the best route for long-term survival.

The three tools for detection are breast self-examination (BSE), mammography, and clinical examinations, although for *early* detection, mammography is far superior. For a complete description of how to do BSE, which should be performed monthly by all women aged 20 and over, see Figures 2-1, 2-2, and 2-3. The guidelines for breast cancer detection are given in the box on page 32.

Mammography has been a source of controversy for many years, with arguments over radiation exposure, insurance coverage of the cost, and whether yearly screening in women under the age of 50 detects enough cancer to justify its cost. As indicated in the chart on page 32, yearly mammography for women 40 and over is recommended by the American Cancer Society (ACS). Controversy about yearly screening between the National Cancer Institute and the ACS for women aged 40 to 50 dominated the 1990s, and appears to have been largely resolved. Most radiologists and oncologists recommend that women begin screening mammography in their 40s, and reimbursement guidelines for insurance companies and HMOs seem to have followed suit. Despite complaints from some cancer advocates that mammography equipment is still not sophisticated enough, the X ray is capable of detecting early cancerous changes in the breast years before a lump becomes palpable (able to be felt).

Be sure to schedule your mammogram after your period, so that your breasts will not be tender. Be prepared for some discomfort, as your breasts will be squeezed between two plastic plates to get a correct reading. (See Figure 2-4.) Try to relax. And remember: This is a tool for monitoring your breast health that you should not neglect.

Some women may be worried when they have discharge from one or both nipples. According to breast surgeon Dr. Susan Love, most discharge is nothing to be alarmed about. Interestingly,

---

American Cancer Society Guidelines for Breast Cancer Detection

Breast self-examination: Age 20 and over: monthly

Clinical breast examination: Age 20–39: every 3 years
Age 40 and over: yearly

Mammography: Age 35–39: baseline
Age 40–49: every 1–2 years
Age 50 and over: yearly

Source: The American Cancer Society, Revised 12/90-No. 2088; reprinted by permission.

How to Do Breast Self-Examination

1. Lie down and put a pillow under your right shoulder. Place your right arm behind your head. (See Figure 2-1.)

2. Use the finger pads of your three middle fingers on your left hand to feel for lumps or thickening. Your finger pads are the top third of each finger. (See Figure 2-2.)

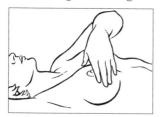

FIGURE 2-1

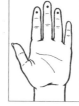

FIGURE 2-2

3. Press firmly enough to know how your breast feels. If you're not sure how hard to press, ask your health care provider. Or try to copy the way your health care provider uses his or her finger pads during a breast exam. Learn what your breast feels like most of the time. A firm ridge in the lower curve of each breast is normal.

4. Move your finger pads over your breast in a me-thodical pattern. One example of such a pattern is the inset Figure 2-3. Another way would be to move around your breast in concentric circles. Choose which way is best for you, and do it the same way each time. Using this set pattern will **FIGURE 2-3** help you to make sure that you've gone over the entire breast area and to remember how your breast feels. Don't forget to also check your armpits for any lumps or thickening.

Source: American Cancer Society; reprinted by permission.

Other tips: For added safety, you might want to check your breast while standing in front of a mirror right after you do your breast self-exam each month. See if there are any changes in the way your breasts look: dimpling of the skin, changes in the nipple, or redness and swelling. Some women choose to do a breast self-exam while in the shower. Your soapy hands glide well over your wet skin, making it easy to check how your breasts feel.

menopause is one of the times when more discharge appears. According to Dr. Love, you should consult your doctor if:

- discharge is spontaneous—comes out by itself without squeezing; or

- discharge is unilateral—on only one side; or

- discharge is clear and sticky, like egg white, or if the fluid is bloody.

Only about 4 percent of these types of discharge are actually caused by invasive cancer. Various problems with the breast ducts, such as wartlike growths, or a cancer called *intraductal carcinoma in situ* (which means the cancer is contained and has not spread) can be responsible.

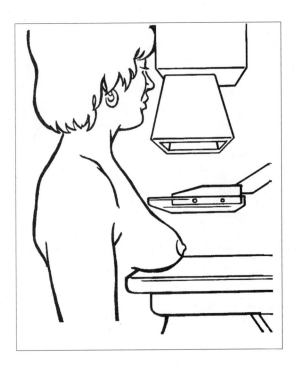

Figure 2-4   *Source:* American Cancer Society.

Let's Talk About Weight

Being obese, or 20 percent over the recommended weight range for your age group, is an independent risk factor for heart disease. In other words, all other factors being equal, a woman who is obese is much more likely to develop cardiovascular disease than a woman who is not obese. Of course, being overweight is not the only indicator of possible heart disease. Even thin women can have familial hypercholesterolemia (abnormally high cholesterol levels). So eating right and taking medication are important for these women. A thin frame can also make a person more susceptible to bone disease. In general, though, women in middle age struggle with extra pounds. If you are more than 20 percent over the normal range, losing weight sensibly can better your chances of long-term quality of life.

Researchers tell us that as we age it becomes harder to lose weight. That's probably no surprise to you! Taking off a quick 10 pounds might have been easy in your 20s, but after 35, it's a much more arduous process for most women. And from what we now know about the dangers of yo-yo dieting (the lose-gain-lose-gain treadmill), especially for the heart, that's probably just as well. Appendix C contains some recommendations from the American Heart Association and from the National Academy of Sciences for eating programs to help prevent heart disease and cancer. Women also diet for reasons other than health, though, and this section will help you frame a context for your attitudes about weight and dieting.

As women move into menopause, they'll be confronted with their own and society's notions about aging. Naturally enough, you may find yourself scrutinizing your body more as you approach 50. Are you generally happy with your body and the way it looks? Whose standards are you using when you judge your appearance?

Is Dieting the Answer?

Just as the perimenopause is an opportune time to reevaluate your health risks, it may also be a good time to scrutinize your values about weight and appearance. Women in middle age may be able to look more realistically at their goals for their appearance, say experts who specialize in treating eating disorders. If you're about to embark on an eating program, it may be helpful to look at the criteria in the box on page 37 ("Readiness to Diet") as a way to assess whether you are setting yourself up for success or failure.

Set Realistic Goals

The norms for average weight are also changing. Although the range of weights in proportion to heights has been adjusted upward, there is a fair amount of controversy about the Metropolitan Life height and weight tables, notes Edward Abramson. Consult Appendix D for current height and weight standards from the U.S. Department of Agriculture to see what the range for your age is. If losing weight has been a problem for you, it may be helpful to relax your standards a bit.

"If someone has a lengthy history of being overweight, it's less likely that they will somehow manage to get themselves down to what the charts say ideally they should be," Abramson notes. "But there is reason to believe that mild to moderate weight losses are useful in terms of improving health even if the net effect still leaves you considerably above what it says in the charts. So if you're 80 pounds overweight and you lose 30 pounds, that's still a significant improvement.

"I also think it's helpful to have a target and a succession of goals. So if you think you ideally would like to lose 80 pounds, rather than set your goal at losing 80 pounds, maybe the goal ought to be to lose 20 pounds and then see how that goes; and then if you like, set another 20-pound weight loss goal.

"And in terms of coming up with a number, I always think it's helpful to have a range," advises Abramson. "So it may make sense to set a goal which will improve your health even though aesthetically you are still not too happy about it."

Readiness to Diet

1. Get a handle on emotional eating. "If you're still using food to deal with emotional stressors, then you've got a strike against you when you start your diet," counsels California State University, Chico, psychologist and author Edward Abramson. "Sooner or later you are going to encounter an emotional stressor, and if your typical pattern is to run to the refrigerator, then that's the end of the diet."

2. Decide for whom you are dieting. Are you dieting to make your husband or your doctor happy? Ideally, *you* should be the person you're trying to please, and hopefully, the reason you want to lose weight is so that you'll be healthier.

3. Examine the current stress level in your life. "Dieting is effortful and requires that you be able to focus on it," Abramson points out. "If you are going through a divorce or are having a lot of difficulty with teenage kids or you've got a new job or some other upheaval is taking place, then you probably shouldn't diet."

4. Plan on increasing energy expenditure. Especially as you get older, there's a limit on how much you can restrict your caloric intake. And in view of the critical role played by calcium for aging bones, it's not a good idea to cut out all dairy products. "Overweight people shudder when I use the word 'exercise,'" says Abramson, "so I try not to use it. But there are noncompetitive ways of increasing energy expenditure where you don't have to feel out of place. You don't have to go to aerobics classes with 18-year-olds. Get together with a friend and walk or bicycle. Do something that isn't competitive, something that doesn't require any particular athletic skill. It doesn't even have to be strenuous; that's one thing that's been demonstrated to my satisfaction—the psychological benefits of exercise, in terms of self-esteem and mood, occur even if you don't get the aerobic benefit."

Source: Edward Abramson, Ph.D., California State University, Chico, author of *Emotional Eating.*

Adjusting Image to Reality

Look at Marilyn Monroe's size versus Cher's or Julia Roberts' size and you can see how overly restrictive current standards of beauty have become.

Edward Abramson, Ph.D., California State University, Chico

Many women tend to judge themselves harshly when it comes to weight and appearance. That's hard to avoid in a culture such as ours. Advertisers promise eternal good looks if only we use a certain "age-denying makeup" or try the latest slimming milkshake. Even self-confident career women can find themselves buying into the idea of being judged by appearances rather than accomplishment. It's hard to resist those messages, but if a woman is going to be happy with herself, resist them she must.

If you haven't come to terms with your appearance, menopause could make simmering conflicts worse. It's already apparent that the number of "boomer" women in midlife have made marketing inroads on this score. Witness articles in *Mirabella* heralding the return of the curvaceous body or in the magazine *Mode,* which features big, bosomy, and ample-hipped models. Despite all these healthy signs, however, chances are you haven't escaped the cultural and advertising messages that skinnier is sexier. By the time they reach their teens, most American females have internalized these messages and have learned to be at war with their bodies. Compiling a personal assessment of how you view your body can be another important component of good preventive care. Just as you want to be sure you're getting the right amounts of exercise and nutrients, accepting your body is another way of being good to yourself.

In her private practice work, University of Cincinnati psychologist Ann Kearney-Cooke uses guided imagery to help women go back through time and explore key events in forming their body image histories.

Then she trains women to "really look inside for direction. Instead of always looking outside your body to figure out what to eat or what to do or what you should look like, place the compass for direction inside your own body," she advises.

"Every body has a history, and that history affects the way you feel about your body," Kearney-Cooke continues. "If your body image history is that you've always hated your body, or felt it was dirty or not good enough, this [menopause] is just another time when you'll get stirred up and struggle. Your body becomes a battleground."

In addition to guided imagery, Kearney-Cooke assigns field work to the women in her groups. The assignment may be to go to the mall or out in the neighborhood and just observe other people and how they look. These women "often come back surprised," reports Kearney-Cooke. After spending some time observing regular people, many women in her group realize that they've carried distorted images of the "ideal" woman around in their heads. "They say to me, 'You know, I didn't realize how much I've distorted [my image of myself], thinking that there's something wrong with me. I looked around and saw that if you were trying to compare yourself to the ideal, there isn't one: The norm isn't the norm.'"

Kearney-Cooke finds that once women are freed of external standards of appearance, they begin to focus on what matters. That often means setting new goals, such as returning to school, trying new options in employment, becoming an entrepreneur, or simply taking up a favorite hobby, like singing or photography. "Once people understand why they have made their bodies a battleground and begin to free themselves up, they will often try new things and begin to see that they have new options," she says.

Good Health and Your Comfort Level

If you've been conscientious about your health, this chapter may help you to fine-tune your health program and focus on areas that will become increasingly important with menopause. If this is a new area for you, don't feel compelled to "redo" yourself and your health program all at once. The information in this chapter is offered as a way to take a look at where you are now and where you might be able to make improvements.

Now you're probably curious about just what's in store with those infamous menopausal symptoms. Chapter 3 gives you the signs to look for.

Best Resources

Books

Dr. Susan Love's Breast Book, 3d edition, by Susan M. Love, M.D., with Karen Lindsey. Perseus Book Group, Cambridge, Mass., 2000; paperback, 632 pages; $20.00.

This is one of the finest women's health books in bookstores today. It is thorough, well-researched, and written in a straightforward and accessible manner. The book covers all aspects of breast health, including options for women diagnosed with breast cancer. Its compassionate tone combined with a wealth of knowledge make this book a must for every woman's health library.

Emotional Eating, by Edward Abramson, Ph.D. Jossey-Bass, San Francisco, 1998; paperback, 208 pages; $19.00.

Written by a professor of psychology at California State University, Chico, who is also a psychologist in private practice, this book gives the reader real tools to use in breaking the cycle of emotional eating. The book's self-assessment questionnaires and accessible writing style can help you understand your patterns of emotional eating and confront your own negative messages, thus clearing the way for greater self-understanding and control.

Women and Heart Disease: What You Can Do to Stop the Number-One Killer of American Women, by Edward B. Diethrich, M.D., and Carol Cohan. Times Books, New York, 1994; paperback, 320 pages; $10.00.

This book, written by the medical director of the Arizona Heart Institute and Foundation with coauthor Carol Cohan, supplies the grim facts and figures about women and heart disease. It also provides a comprehensive discussion of heart disease symptoms, as well as those specific to women, so that we can demand appropriate screening even if our doctors neglect it.

Perimenopause: Changes in Women's Health After 35, by James E. Huston, M.D., and L. Darlene Lanka, M.D. New Harbinger Publications, Inc., Oakland, Calif., 1997; paperback, 394 pages; $16.95.

Dr. Lanka is the director for women's health at Kaiser Permanente, Walnut Creek, California, and an assistant clinical professor at the University of San Francisco.

Pamphlets and Newsletters

"Before You Start Your Next Diet . . ." takes a critical look at the societal pressures to diet and helps the reader find realistic expectations for her own weight loss. This and other pamphlets are distributed by NAAFA (National Association to Advance Fat Acceptance), P.O. Box 188620, Sacramento, CA 95818.

Women's Health Letter
P.O. Box 467939
Atlanta, GA 31146-7939
(800) 728-2288 or
(770) 399-5617

This eight-page monthly newsletter covers all aspects of women's health, with a special emphasis on nutrition. "News Briefs" offers summaries of relevant medical studies, and "Woman to Woman" answers readers' specific health questions. Editor-in-chief and nutrition expert Nan Kathryn Fuchs, Ph.D., offer thought-provoking articles each month. Not all the articles are about midlife health, but there's always lots from which to pick and choose. A year's subscription is $39; two years' worth of newsletters is offered at $77.

Associations

Arizona Heart Institute and Foundation
2632 North 20th Street
Phoenix, AZ 85006
(602) 266-2200
www.azheart.com

More information on heart disease in women, along with answers to your questions and helpful brochures, are available by calling the Arizona Heart Institute and Foundation. Edward B. Diethrich, M.D., the director of the institute, is an expert on heart disease in women. His book, *Women and Heart Disease: What You Can Do to Stop the Number One Killer of American Women,* is available through the institute if you cannot find it elsewhere.

American Cancer Society
(800) ACS-2345
(800) 227-2345
www.cancer.org

The ACS Web site is an excellent source of information on the prevention, diagnosis, and treatment of all cancers. Click on "cancer" to get to the "Breast Cancer Resource Center." When you call their toll-free number, the American Cancer Society (ACS) can provide information regarding cancer prevention and treatment. Calls are picked up regionally, so you needn't be concerned about time zones. Nutritional pamphlets such as "Mother Was Right" contain basic guidelines on cancer prevention diets.

CHAPTER THREE

Is This It? The Signs and Symptoms of Menopause

I wasn't really sure what was happening at first. I had what I thought was a hot flash right around my 50th birthday. I just got a little hot in the face and perspired. It wasn't much. But about two months after that, it started happening almost every day and sometimes at night, so I went to my doctor for a blood test. When the results came back and she told me I was in menopause, I felt like having a glass of champagne!

Jane, 50

I took estrogen for years following my complete hysterectomy, which happened when I was in my late 40s. But I got breast cancer when I was 58 and underwent a radical mastectomy. I've been cancer-free for 12 years, but I had to give up taking estrogen. Now here I am, 70 years old, and *still* having hot flashes. I do notice that I get more of them during hot weather, if I'm more physically active, and when I'm under a lot of stress. So if I'm able to tailor my habits ahead of time to those events, I can sort of lessen the discomfort.

Marilyn, 70

Two women, two totally different experiences with hot flashes. For one, hot flashes are an almost joyous marker of a life transition. For another, they're a nuisance she'd rather not be dealing with. How do hot flashes happen? Why are they one of the most universal signs of impending menopause?

For both Jane and Marilyn, as well as for the majority of menopausal women, the appearance of hot flashes is related to the body's adjustment to changes in the hormone system: among them, dropping estrogen and progesterone levels and fluctuations in FSH (follicle stimulating hormone) and LH (luteinizing hormone). Not all women experience signs of estrogen deprivation, however. A minority may even experience excess estrogen, one of the signs of which is dysfunctional bleeding. (If you have unusually heavy and unpredictable uterine bleeding, you need to be seen by a doctor, since this can also indicate serious conditions such as uterine fibroids or precancerous growth of the uterine lining.)

Will you experience hot flashes, and if you do, what will they be like? How long does it take to "get through" menopause? This chapter describes the process that triggers menopause, a chain of events that are only part of your body's reproductive continuum. Charts, lists, and women's stories will illustrate the variety of physical responses during menopause. You'll find out whom you should consult (see "Finding the Best Allies" on page 55) and which test can best define your menopausal status (see box, "Are You in Menopause?" on page 49).

Also in this chapter, you'll become familiar with the range of menopausal signs. Then, in Chapter 4, you'll be introduced to a whole variety of approaches—both conventional and alternative—for dealing with your symptoms.

How to View Your Symptoms

Some women have trouble telling whether their menopause has begun. They may not have hot flashes or other discomforts, or their symptoms may be erratic and fleeting. For other women, there is no doubt—symptoms literally wake them up at night and disrupt routines during the day. Menopause is not an illness or a disease, as was thought for centuries. But when symptoms become severe, there are times when a woman may feel as if something is going terribly wrong with her body.

It may be helpful to look back at the time when you and your peers experienced *menarche*, or first menstruation. As preadolescents, your bodies all responded differently when you got your periods. Now, as then, we'll each have different responses to menopause, and different reactions to menopausal symptoms. One thing's for certain: We don't have to operate in the dark. Thanks to more attention in the press and the political arena, which led in part to the establishment of the Women's Health Initiative, menopause will become better understood with each coming year. The scientific literature is already immense: Scientists are studying everything from bone health and hot flashes to sexual functioning and gastric emptying (the time it takes for the stomach to empty after a meal) in the menopausal woman.

Understanding menopause becomes easier when you look at it as the completion of a cycle that began when you were in utero. That's when the primitive cells that are to become egg follicles start to grow. Then, between 9 and 14 years of age, you probably experienced menarche, the beginning of your menstrual periods. When you began menstruating, you had a visible marker of your body's readiness to procreate.

The menstrual cycle is complicated, based on feedback mechanisms between the pituitary gland and hypothalamus in the brain. Messages are conveyed via the hormones FSH (follicle stimulating hormone) and LH (luteinizing hormone), signaling the ovary to ripen egg follicles already within the organ. When an egg follicle begins to mature, it in turn stimulates the ovary to produce estrogens, which are carried to target organs like the uterus and the breasts. These organs have estrogen receptors that allow the hormone compound to attach and then act on the cells to encourage growth. Before a woman's period, her breasts tend to swell and her uterine lining gets thicker in anticipation of the egg being fertilized and having a suitable place to be implanted. Progesterone, secreted by the sac (corpus luteum) that forms where the egg was released, also plays a role in this process. When the egg is not fertilized, progesterone triggers the sloughing off of the enriched uterine lining as a menstrual period.

With menopause, different sets of markers signal that these features of the reproductive process are coming to a close.

Your Ovaries Slow Down

From the time of your first period until your 40s, your ovaries produce estrogen in response to monthly follicle maturation. When I refer to "estrogen" in the text, I am using a general term that includes examples of a whole class of compounds that produce female sexual effects. Estrogens are found everywhere in nature and function, in general, as growth hormones. All estrogens have the same effect—stimulating growth—but not the same potency. The most potent naturally occurring human estrogen, *estradiol,* causes the uterine lining to thicken before a period. Most of the estrogen produced by the ovaries is either estradiol or *estrone*; the former is more potent than the latter, and estrone is also manufactured in fat cells and other peripheral cells by conversion of the precursor steroid, *androstenedione.* A third type, *estriol,* is produced as a byproduct from estradiol and estrone metabolism and is primarily important during pregnancy.

Both estrogen and progesterone are responsible for the monthly menstrual cycle and both are produced using precursor *androgenic* (male) hormones. During her reproductive years, a woman's ovaries produce more estrogen than testosterone. As menopause nears, the estrogen level declines while the androgenic level stays about the same. Lacking former levels of estrogen to counteract them, such androgenic effects as hair growth on the face and oily skin may begin to crop up during the years right before menopause in some women.

You are born with a huge supply of potential eggs—over half a million. Over time, that number decreases as some are reabsorbed back into the ovarian lining. In your lifetime, about 400 to 450 eggs will mature and be released from your ovaries. As you age, the number of eggs available for release diminishes. From about age 40 on, most women will experience at least some cycles that are *anovulatory* (without the release of an egg). As that happens, the levels of estrogen and progesterone will fluctuate, and a woman's periods will start to change.

Then, in her mid-40s, as a woman gets closer to the time of menopause, she becomes perimenopausal. The period of time from perimenopause to postmenopause, which varies with each woman, can take from 5 to 10 years. Women who have complete hysterectomies, when both the ovaries and uterus are removed, or oophorectomies, removal of ovaries only, experience an abrupt surgical menopause. For this type of menopause, there is no transition.

Joann, an active 57-year-old who takes estrogen daily, recalls, "My hot flashes hit me with a bang the very day after my surgery. There was no fooling around. My doctor prescribed estrogen and I was glad to begin the therapy. I've been in great health ever since!"

The Climacteric Can Take 20 Years

The diagnosis of a natural menopause is, by definition, retrospective. A woman is menopausal when she has not menstruated for 12 months (some experts say it can be as little as 6 months, but these are in the minority.) Still, as one woman pointed out to me, "I'm confused—as soon as the event is confirmed, does that mean I'm immediately *postmenopausal?*" Precise measurement of beginnings and endings are not useful during the menopausal transition, because your body's changes are actually occurring on a continuum, not a start-and-stop basis. That's why you may also hear the term *climacteric,* because it encompasses a whole spectrum of changes from decreased fertility, to cessation of menstruation, to the manifestations of estrogen deprivation, such as tissue atrophy. For American women, menopause usually occurs between ages 48 and 55; the average age can be anywhere between 50 and 52. Expert opinion varies on the "exact" age, precisely because it is a transition and not one single event.

A full decade before you become menopausal, changes are happening in your body that begin to set the stage for the transition from reproductive to nonreproductive states. A good

Age Span of the Climacteric

Perimenopausal	Menopausal	Postmenopausal
⊢—— Age 40 ——————	— Age 50—————	—Age 55–60——⊣
Ovulation decreases	Hot flashes, vaginal changes	Cessation of menses
Menstruation infrequent		

percentage of women—from 40 to 58 percent—start experiencing hot flashes in the two-year period before cessation of menstruation. Menstruation at this time is likely to be erratic. During this segment of changes, a woman is considered perimenopausal. *Climacteric* is often used as an all-inclusive term to denote the whole spectrum of pre- to postmenopausal changes, although some sources use the term interchangeably with *perimenopause*.

Menopausal and Perimenopausal Symptoms

As noted in Chapter 1, the exception is often the rule when it comes to menopausal symptoms. In a comprehensive review of journal articles on menopause, however, Gail A. Greendale, M.D., and Howard L. Judd, M.D., both of UCLA, note that the transitional menstrual pattern is typically characterized by long intervals between periods interspersed with short intervals between periods. In other words, your periods are no longer regular and predictable. This is because the remaining egg follicles in your ovaries do not mature consistently. Your cycles may be ovulatory, with a mid-cycle estrogen surge followed by progesterone release, or anovulatory, with corresponding rise and fall of estrogen levels without progesterone secretion (which has to come from the ripened egg case). Fewer follicles are available, so less estrogen is produced.

In an effort to get the ovaries going, the pituitary sends more FSH, the hormone released to stimulate egg maturation, to the ovaries. A high level of FSH is the true marker that you are in menopause. Although some physicians maintain that measuring estrogen levels in the blood and vaginal tissues can also indicate whether a woman is in menopause, the FSH is considered the standard test. (See Table 3-1, "Tests to Determine Menopausal Status," on page 50.) In addition, an estrogen test can also be skewed because of estrogen production from indirect sources, such as conversion of fatty tissues to estrone. The estrone will continue to circulate in your blood and furnish a supply of estrogen, although it is a weaker hormone than estradiol. Some research has shown that women whose bodies generate more estrone may have a milder menopausal transition.

Where Do You Fit In?

Where will you fit on this continuum? Although you cannot predict which signs of menopause you will have, or their frequency and severity, researchers have begun to notice some indicators:

- Women who are overweight tend to have fewer hot flashes. Researchers think this is because their bodies metabolize some additional estrogens from fat tissues, so the estrogen withdrawal is somewhat mitigated.

- If your periods are coming closer together (26 days or less) during the perimenopause, you may go through menopause slightly sooner.

- If you've been a smoker, you will most likely experience menopause about two years before the average age of 50.

- If you've had an abdominal hysterectomy (removal of the uterus only), the blood supply to your ovaries may have been compromised and you may also go through an earlier menopause.

- Living at high altitudes is also associated with an earlier menopause.

Are You in Menopause?

According to reproductive endocrinologist Paul Stumpf, M.D., of the Jersey Shore Medical Center, "The FSH [follicle stimulating hormone] is the most useful test for diagnosing menopause. You would think that you could diagnose menopause by measuring the estrogen level, but the problem with that is that estrogen is cleared pretty rapidly from the body. It has a half-life of about one hour. So you could measure it at a given point in time and it might be high, but the total exposure to estrogen might be inadequate. The FSH is a test that reflects the brain's exposure to estrogen. It gives you a marker for what the total exposure to estrogen is most of the time." See Table 3-1.

TABLE 3-1   Tests to Determine Menopausal Status

Blood Level of FSH	Status
Under 40	Not menopausal
40–100	In a transition period
Over 100	Through the menopause

Additional Tests Used by Practitioners
Vaginal smears
Estrogen levels in blood

- About 1 percent of women go through premature menopause (before the age of 40).

Your menopause may not be very eventful—that is, you may simply stop menstruating one month and never resume. Chances are, though, that you will experience at least some of the signs of menopause. These fall into two categories: changes you notice, and changes you may not notice (but of which you should take note).

The Changes You Notice

As you already know, estrogen affects many organs in the body. Target organs, those that have specific receptors for estrogen, include the uterus, ovaries, fallopian tubes, vagina, bladder, urethra, and the breasts. In addition, estrogens also affect the skin (causing cells that bind with it to take up more fluid, thus making the skin puffier), the central nervous system (most notably the pituitary, hypothalamus, and spinal cord), the gastrointestinal system (colon, pancreas, and liver), the adrenal gland, the circulatory system (heart and arteries), and the skeletal system. What follows are some of the signs your body starts exhibiting when estrogen levels fall and these target organs are no longer exposed to the same levels of the hormone.

Common signs of menopause

The most noticed symptom of the climacteric is the hot flash (also called flush, because women report a flushed feeling about the face and neck). Some physicians and researchers group hot flashes together with sweats (mostly occurring at night) as *vasomotor complaints*. Various explanations for the cause of hot flashes have been put forth over the past decades. Documented elevated levels of LH (produced mostly during ovulation) during hot flashes were once thought to be the cause. Current theory proposes that certain brain chemicals called *catecholamines* and *opiates* may mediate hot flashes. It's now believed that the hypothalamus, one of the glands affected by estradiol withdrawal, somehow releases a trigger substance that results in thermoregulatory instability. The body's signals get mixed, triggering a warming and sweating sequence, in an effort to stabilize what it perceives as a change in body temperature.

Whatever the cause of the hot flash, it can be mild, moderate, or severe. Estimates of how many women have hot flashes vary, from 70 percent in some studies to as high as 85 percent in others. Somewhere within the two-year time frame around their last period, at least 40 to 58 percent of women will experience hot flashes. Between one-quarter and one-half of these women may have flashes for longer than five years.

The average hot flash lasts 3.3 minutes, with some as short as half a minute and some as long as one hour. Although they don't know how hot flashes happen, researchers can measure changes in skin and core temperature, as well as resistance by the moisture in the skin.

> *My hot flashes come on in the space of a minute. First I feel a slight warmth in my chest area. Then my face and scalp start to feel real hot. If someone's in the room, they tell me my face is getting red. I feel the perspiration coming, and that's when I head for the bathroom. I pat my face dry with a slightly damp towel, loosen my collar, and comb my hair. Then I'm fine, until the next one!* —Lydia, 53

Lydia's hot flashes appear to follow almost a classic pattern. Many women report that they have an "aura" or premonition right before the onset of the hot flash. Most often, perspiring accompanies the hot flash. Sweating can also occur by itself without a hot flash. Witness Nicky, 55, who wakes up drenched in perspiration and has to change not only her nightgown, but her sheets as well. One episode of the comic strip "For Better or for Worse," by Lynn Johnston, playfully illustrated the phenomenon. The wife tosses and turns all night, unable to get cool or comfortable. Her husband is kept awake, too, and remarks to an office worker the next morning, "I think I'm going through the change of wife." No wonder that, for some couples, as sex therapist Wendy Schain, Ph.D., notes, "Menopause is a family affair"!

Keeping in mind estrogen's target organs, other noticeable and common menopausal changes include those in the genital area. Estrogen depletion causes the pH balance of the vaginal mucosa to change, so the lining of your vagina becomes thinner and may lubricate less well. This can lead to more vaginal infections. In some women, the loss of estrogen may actually cause the outer skin of the vagina to become cracked and to bleed. The vagina may shorten, and the cervix can eventually become closed and migrate upward into the cervical canal, making a Pap smear difficult to obtain.

Changes to the urinary tract are also common. These tissues are estrogen-sensitive, as are the skin, vagina, breasts, bones, heart, and pituitary system. As the body shifts away from the monthly dose of body-produced estrogen and progesterone, women may notice urinary tract changes: more infections, more frequent urination, or more uncontrolled urination. Bladder tone is dependent on estrogen, and with its loss, the muscles become more lax. This effect, combined with the stresses produced from childbearing, can produce stress incontinence. This means that a woman loses a small bit of urine when she coughs, sneezes, runs, or laughs. If not treated, this can become quite a problem. It can be handled in a number of ways, including hormone therapy, strengthening the pelvic floor muscles with Kegel exercises, or other natural and/or behavioral remedies (see Chapter 4).

Less common, or atypical, signs

There are a whole range of additional signs and symptoms associated with menopause. Some of these may be caused by menopause and some may simply be happening coincidentally to it. For instance, headaches often increase in menopausal and postmenopausal women. Some scientists believe they're estrogen-related, since estrogen acts almost like an opiate in the brain.

Many other changes have been noted by women during menopause and cover a wide spectrum, including tenseness; heart palpitations; irritability; a feeling of "pins and needles," especially in the extremities; a condition called "restless legs"; dizziness; tiredness; tiredness on waking; depression; forgetfulness; lack of energy; shortness of breath; lack of self-confidence; insomnia; muscle pain (myalgia) or joint pain (arthralgia); itching labia; and vaginal discharge.

It should be noted that although these complaints have been reported by women in menopause, it is important to make sure that they are not symptomatic of another medical condition. For instance, heart palpitations and shortness of breath, if occurring together, can be symptoms of underlying heart disease. By the same token, tiredness, insomnia, and lack of self-confidence can be signs of clinical depression, and you should consult a psychologist or other mental health professional for help with that.

The Changes You May Not Notice

Your body won't signal you with all its responses to menopause right away. The other, long-term results of estrogen loss will be covered more fully in Chapter 6. The invisible or silent concerns arising after menopause are excessive bone loss and proclivity toward heart disease. These heart, vascular system, and bone loss problems do create certain signs, and you can remain aware of them by following recommended checkup schedules. (See "Your Before and During HRT Checklist" on page 79.)

Keeping Track

Do you need to take note of each and every one of these menopause-related changes? If you're not bothered by vaginal dryness or tiredness, or if they occur only occasionally, it may not be important to track their frequency. But keeping a record of the changes in your period is definitely a good idea. Remember that nuisance question the nurse always asks when you go for your yearly gynecological visit: "When was the date of your last period?" This question will become even more important as you enter the climacteric. It's simple enough to devise a method for keeping track. I keep a small, wallet-sized calendar in my purse in which I record simple notes, such as "23rd day, spotting," or "27th day, began period, 2 days late."

Many of the menopause books out now, notably those by Drs. Notelovitz and Utian (see "Best Resources" at the end of Chapter 1), have examples of excellent menopausal symptom diaries, and you may find them helpful. Make the process as easy as possible so that it doesn't require much effort to include it in your daily, weekly, or monthly routine. Table 3-2 is an excerpt from Rosetta Reitz's *Menopause: A Positive Approach*, showing you how she dealt with tracking her own signs and symptoms. You may want to borrow from each record-keeping method you read about and devise your own simple system.

TABLE 3-2   Menopause Menstrual Record

Date of Period	Amount of Flow	Days from Last Period
50½ years old		
February 12	4 days	29
March 8	4 days	25
April	no period	
May	no period	
June 21	3 days	105
July 21	3½ days, heavy	31
August	no period	
September	no period	
51 years old		
October	no period	
November 15	4 days	118
December	no period	

Source: Rosetta Reitz, *Menopause: A Positive Approach*, New York: Penguin Books, 1977, p. 23.

A Plan of Action

Now that you're familiar with the constellation of possible menopausal symptoms, what do you do about them? You may want to visit your doctor now to get a checkup, have some blood levels drawn, and in general discuss possible plans of action.

If you've begun talks with your doctor before the climacteric, and feel comfortable with the physician, chances are you're already discussing menopausal changes during your regular visits.

Interrupted sleep, interrupted concentration, sweating, and flushing all can add up to making you uncomfortable and irritable. Use these signs and symptoms as an incentive to seek the right professional, one who understands the complexity of the climacteric and is willing to treat you as an individual. Keeping track of signs and symptoms can be helpful to your health care practitioner as well, providing clues to your progress and alerting the doctor to any possible other conditions that may warrant testing.

I was recently reminded that trying to second-guess your symptoms and diagnose your condition can be way off target. Figuring that I was entering menopause (frequent insomnia, weight gain, some depression, and depressed sex drive), I was set to consult my ob/gyn to "start the talk" about HRT. In the meantime, I had visited my family practice physician, who's a very thorough and up-to-date doctor. She suggested I have a blood panel drawn since it had been a while. To my surprise, the test revealed that I was not in menopause (FSH levels were still within range) but that I did have hypothyroidism. Many of the symptoms listed above are also signs of an underactive thyroid. Coincidentally, this is quite common in middle-aged women. While my hypothyroidism is being treated, I still can look forward to going into menopause!

Finding the Best Allies

You don't necessarily need a "menopause expert" to treat you as you go through the climacteric. For general health problems, even those of menopause, you could consult your general family practitioner, internist, or personal ob/gyn specialist. Or, you may prefer someone with a specialty in reproductive endocrinology, a physician who is board certified to treat problems of the reproductive hormone system.

When evaluating your present doctor, or a new one, consider these issues:

- Does the physician listen to your complaints and answer your questions to your satisfaction?
- Does the office staff answer any additional questions you may have?
- Does the physician appear to be aware of the latest information on menopause and women's health?
- Is the physician willing to change therapies and/or regimens if you are having trouble?
- Is the physician's gender important to you? If so, make sure that you choose a female gynecologist, for instance, if you feel most comfortable with a woman. On the other hand, perhaps the way you are treated is more important and gender is secondary. Make sure you listen to your feelings.
- Is the physician open to alternative treatments you may suggest? For instance, if you consult a chiropractor or an acupuncturist, will the physician be offended or condemn your actions?
- If the practitioner is in alternative medicine, do you have reliable ways to check credentials? (See suggestions in Chapter 4 for choosing a chiropractor and choosing an herbalist.)
- Do you have the resources or private insurance coverage to pay for this doctor? If you belong to an HMO (health maintenance organization) or PPO (preferred provider organization), do you have the ability to pick your own doctor(s)? Consult the following "Best Resources" section for more suggestions regarding how to find the right doctor for you at this time of life.

Best Resources

Books

Understanding Menopause: Answers and Advice for Women in the Prime of Life, by Janine O'Leary Cobb. NAL-Dutton, New York, 1993; paperback, 336 pages; $11.00.

Written by one of the most respected women's health care advocates, this book covers medical and nonmedical remedies and explains what menopause is and what to expect. The information is spliced together with anecdotes from her and other women's experiences. Well written, using the same friendly and accessible tone that makes the same author's *A Friend Indeed* newsletter so well received.

The New Ourselves, Growing Older—Women Aging with Knowledge and Power, by Paula Brown Doress, Diana Laskin Siegal, and the Midlife and Older Women Book Project, in cooperation with the Boston Women's Health Collective. Touchstone Books, New York, 1994; paperback, 531 pages; $20.00.

The most recent edition of this weighty book contains a greeting from the authors: "We welcome baby boomers to the promise of many more fulfilling years ahead." With chapter and section titles such as "Aging Well" and "Living with Ourselves and Others as We Age," the book takes a comprehensive social, political, economical, and medical look at all aspects of midlife and older women's health. Political analyses sometimes get in the way of sorting through hard medical data, but on the whole the book is a supportive and very informative one.

Additional Sources of Menopausal Care

Look for group practices in obstetrics and gynecology with a stated policy of treating menopausal women.

Contact the nearest university teaching hospital or medical school for your geographic area, and call the departments of ob/gyn and/or geriatrics to find out if there are clinics available for midlife women. Additional travel may be worthwhile to seek second opinions and consultations.

Contact the
North American Menopause Society
P.O. Box 94527
Cleveland, OH 44101
(440) 442-7550 phone
(440) 442-2660 fax
E-mail: info@menopause.org
www.menopause.org

Founded in 1989 by Wulf H. Utian, M.D., Ph.D., a noted expert on menopause and author of several books on midlife women's health, this nonprofit multidisciplinary professional organization is devoted to promoting the understanding of menopause among health care professionals and consumers. The Web site offers information for both professionals and consumers. One valuable service offers lists of physicians specializing in menopause according to geographic area.

CHAPTER FOUR

The Physical Effects of Menopause: Managing Your Symptoms

I've become so disgusted trying to deal with my symptoms, that if you told me right now you had some sort of tea made from a weird root that would take away the hot flashes, I'd probably go out and try it!

> *Sharon, 52, who has had to temporarily discontinue HRT due to undiagnosed heavy bleeding*

My metabolism went out of whack. I couldn't control my weight no matter what I did. And I got sort of thick in the middle. And my skin got so dry. What really got to me was the dryness. So I went on Premarin and whatever the little orange one is—Provera. . . . But I did get some breakthrough bleeding, and the doctor said, "No problem, that's common, especially in the beginning." But it continued for about a year. . . . I had three pelvic exams and they all said my uterus was just perfectly normal. But you don't take crazy risks like that so I had an endometrial biopsy and it was normal. But the bleeding continued.

The first week I went off estrogen, I lost 12 pounds. And you know 12 pounds in a week is water—I wasn't fat, I was bloated. I tried eating a yam [a plant source of progesterone] a day, but I got too sick of yams. I believe there have to be other methods and certainly there has to be another form of estrogen that is not made out of horse urine.

Penelope, 52

I've been taking estrogen for 20 years now, ever since I had the hysterectomy. For me, it's been great. I've had no problems with it and my energy has been fine. I exercise three times a week, so my weight has never been a problem. For me it was the right thing to do.
    Carol, 56

Perhaps at no other time, except during puberty or pregnancy, is a woman more aware of her body's changes than during menopause. For most women, menopausal changes are noticeable but not totally disruptive. For a minority of women, menopause is asymptomatic, meaning there are no outward signs. For others, symptoms may become intolerable, and finding ways to manage them becomes urgent. The variety of symptoms for which they seek relief include hot flashes, night sweats, vaginal dryness and atrophy (when tissues dry and shrink), as well as many of the more nebulous and nonspecific signs of mental confusion, forgetfulness, moodiness, and depression.

When intolerable symptoms of menopause crop up, we're presented with the challenge of how to handle them. Many remedies are offered, and yet there is no one definitive therapy that will work for every woman. So, where are you most likely to find relief, reliable information, and support? When you ask that question, you often have posed yourself a conundrum.

Medical science offers hormone therapy, which takes care of hot flashes and vaginal atrophy but may present other risks. Long-term studies have yet to be done absolutely establishing that HRT does not cause breast cancer (although, on balance, according to meta-analyses that encompass many studies, the risk is slight). Alternative medicine offers natural hormone compounds but relies on data that often do not appear in peer-reviewed journals and that are not derived from clinical studies recognized by the medical community.

As I approach my own menopause, I, too, wrestle with the glut of conflicting information. I do not foresee an end to this process—of continually sifting through and evaluating information, taking what applies to you, discarding what doesn't, and leaving yourself open for additional information—for some time. We still do not know enough about menopause, we still do not have enough long-term studies that would allow us to more fully understand estrogen's role in the aging process for women. This sets us up for frustration, and understandably so. Women want answers, and they want them now. For my part, I am inclined to rely on studies conducted for publication in peer-reviewed journals.

The argument from some alternative practitioners and consumer advocates is that medical science is too closely allied with pharmaceutical companies that sponsor clinical trials to be objective. Many plant-derived natural compounds are not patented, and drug companies understandably do not want to fund research for something for which they cannot obtain exclusive marketing rights. In their disappointment with Western medicine not having enough answers or having inadequate answers, however, women need to be careful not to place their faith in a remedy just because it is called natural. Selling and marketing products and services are not the province solely of pharmaceutical companies.

In this chapter, I present overviews of several alternative therapies and remedies. Keep in mind that the evidence concerning these remedies is mostly anecdotal, based on descriptions of unmatched individual cases rather than on controlled studies.

Let three principles guide you as you deal with your menopausal symptoms:

First, you are absolutely entitled to a practitioner who not only addresses your concerns but is sympathetic to them. Because so many ob/gyns are male, they may have trouble understanding how significant a side effect is to you. For example, breast tenderness is common when women start HRT. "From a medical point of view," says Paul Stumpf, M.D., of the Jersey Shore Medical Center's menopause clinic, "it's insignificant [because it does not indicate malignancy], but to the patient it's very uncomfortable and very scary." You may decide that you prefer a female doctor. But that's no guarantee your concerns will be heard; empathy is not an exclusive trait of either sex. Many male ob/gyns, especially those who specialize in menopause, can be very sympathetic.

Second, you are absolutely entitled to make your own decision. Information from your doctor and as many other sources as you deem necessary will be your best insurance that you're doing the right thing for your particular circumstances.

Third, the course you set today or next week is not set in stone. If you decide to go on HRT, this will most likely be an evolving process. The first prescription may cause too many side effects; you may decide in two years' time to change therapies or discontinue HRT (which should only be done in concert with talks with your physician). Last year, my baseline bone density scan revealed I was "osteopenic," meaning my bones were not as dense as they should be compared to women my age. Coupled with the fact that my mother has osteoporosis, this revelation compelled me to consider HRT. I began using a combination estrogen/progesterone patch, but two months later during a blood pressure screening, I discovered I had borderline high blood pressure. Within 24 hours of removing the patch, my blood pressure was back to normal. I now follow my nurse practitioner's advice and take Fosamax for my bones.

In this chapter, you'll find suggestions for a variety of ways to cope with menopause symptoms, ranging from standard medical hormone replacement therapy to behavioral remedies focusing on lifestyle and commonsense changes, to alternative healing methods. (Additional considerations about long-term HRT, prescribed to protect the bones and heart into middle age and beyond, will be examined in Chapter 6.)

Where Women Obtain Information

In a Gallup survey sponsored by the North American Menopause Society (NAMS) and reported at the NAMS Fall 1993 annual meeting, pollsters found that a full third of women currently experiencing symptoms did not consult their doctors at all about menopause. And approximately two-thirds of the 833 women questioned (all between the ages of 45 and 60) got their information about menopause from sources other than their doctors: magazine articles and books, friends, television, family members. The explosion of the Internet has accelerated consumer access to health and medical information.

Why are doctors not a main source of information? Women may not feel comfortable bringing up their concerns about menopause in the physician's office. Their doctors may be rushed, unwilling to spend the time required to impart information, and, according to Dr. Stumpf, just plain uncomfortable or inexperienced with the problems of menopause. "The average practicing ob/gyn is not practiced at modifying endocrine therapies very much. There is perhaps more of a rigid perspective on how things ought to be prescribed . . . and, like most other folks, prescribers try to avoid problems or complaints. So when somebody does complain or has a problem or difficulty, it's sometimes easier to just give up than to try to work with the person."

While women in previous generations might have been willing to give up on their therapies (or give up on their doctors!), today's health-conscious women are getting better at asking for information. Now that they are asking questions, most will probably discover that their physicians favor hormone replacement therapy to replenish the estrogens lost during menopause.

The latest revision of the American College of Obstetricians and Gynecologists' *Educational Bulletin* on hormone replacement therapy, dated May 1998, recommends that HRT "should be considered to relieve vasomotor symptoms [hot flashes], genital urinary tract atrophy, and mood and cognitive disturbances, as well as to prevent osteoporosis and cardiovascular disease." In addition, HRT may also be considered to help prevent colon cancer, Alzheimer's disease, and adult tooth loss. The most important indications not to begin HRT include unexplained vaginal bleeding, active liver disease, chronic impaired liver function, recent vascular thrombosis (blood clot), and active breast or uterine cancer.

Now, this bulletin was revised and published prior to publication of the Heart and Estrogen/Progestin Replacement Study (HERS) in August of the same year. To the surprise of many, treatment with oral estrogen plus progestin did not reduce the overall rate of coronary heart disease in postmenopausal women with established coronary illness. And, HRT actually increased the incidence of blood clots and gallbladder disease. Results of this study are causing organizations such as the American Heart Association to rethink recommendations of HRT for older women with coronary disease. "Hormone replacement therapy got grandfathered into our current evidence-based medicine mode," believes Robert Lindsay, M.D., Ph.D., chief of internal medicine at Helen Hayes Regional Bone Center in West Haver-straw, New York, and president of the National Osteoporosis Foundation. "When there have been attempts to do studies that back up what physicians believe from epidemiological studies, it just hasn't worked out. And the classic, of course, was the HERS study, where the effects [of HRT] were not nearly as big as people would have anticipated."

With this much conflicting research, it is probably no surprise that most women, as the Gallup poll showed, do not consider doctors as the first—or last—source of information on menopause and may still balk at such recommendations. According to menopause activist Janine O'Leary Cobb, publisher of *A Friend Indeed* newsletter, physicians just aren't offering their patients much in the way of alternatives.

According to some surveys, most women are afraid of hormone replacement therapy because of the potential risks posed by personal or family health histories. Also, women entering menopause are reluctant to take hormones because of the unknowns, because they don't like taking "medicines," and because they don't want to feel like guinea pigs. And remember, the generation about to enter menopause en masse is the boomer generation, who championed health foods and natural remedies.

Should you try alternative healing methods to get through menopause? Will they provide you with enough health protection later? How can you evaluate an alternative method for its effectiveness? In this chapter, we'll examine what's practical for women and what's not. Sifting through information concerning options that will affect your own body is a challenging process. The more thorough and careful your investigation, the better your chances of making wise choices.

Take the Commonsense Approach

Let's start with the most practical methods first. Unless they feel seriously ill or have warning signs of serious illness, most people prefer to handle symptoms themselves by trying self-help methods. One researcher at Johns Hopkins University who has been studying patient participation in health care decisions has found that when apprised of options and the consequences of treating their condition with surgery or other methods, most patients chose the least invasive therapy.

Although patient decision-making in menopausal women has not been studied yet, my observations from the lectures I've attended and the interviews I've conducted are that most women would prefer the least invasive route for dealing with their symptoms. That's not to say they shouldn't visit their gynecologist for a yearly Pap smear or have definitive FSH blood tests to establish whether they're truly in menopause—or that they shouldn't at least consider the estrogen option for their present health needs (see the section on estrogen later in this chapter) and their future quality of life (see Chapter 6). All things being equal, however, a behavioral or commonsense route might be the best for some women. These methods cost little, except for a commitment to changing your habits, and may yield much. Even so, using such methods may require a great deal of patience. Remember the famous Harvard study that established it takes an average of 21 days to change a habit? That particular research simply involved switching from using a trash can on the right side of one's desk to one on the left side! You're dealing here with a lifetime of habits, good and bad. Knowing which ones to alter and which to retain may take some trial and error, but the payoffs can be well worth the effort.

Practical Tips for Hot Flashes

The most ubiquitous signal of menopause, the hot flash, can also be the most bothersome. Between 75 and 80 percent of menopausal women will experience them, and strategies and remedies abound. Here's a sampling of the range of tips for handling hot flashes from health care practitioners and authors.

- Dress in layered clothing, preferably cotton, since natural fibers allow your skin to breathe. Then when you feel a flash coming on, you can simply shed layers to cool off. Since some flashes are followed by chills, it can be helpful to have a sweater to put back on.

- Limit or eliminate altogether substances that may act as triggers: caffeine; alcohol; hot, spicy foods.

- Drink plenty of water. Keeping well hydrated can help modulate your body temperature.

- Use lighter blankets or a fan near your bed to deal with hot flashes at night.

- Make use of other coping behaviors. Psychological or behavioral coping techniques are getting more attention from the scientific community. For instance, a small study conducted by Robert R. Freedman, Ph.D., a professor of psychiatry at the Lafayette Clinic and Wayne State University School of Medicine in Detroit, found that regular, practiced deep breathing reduced hot flashes by 50 percent in the study's 33 participants. What was interesting about this study is that the other methods—muscle relaxation and biofeedback—produced no change in the hot flash pattern. Women practiced deep breathing for 15 minutes twice a day. They also slowed their breathing as they felt the onset of a hot flash, thus lessening its intensity. It is thought that deep, slow abdominal breaths (6 to 8 a minute instead of the usual 14 to 16) help to prevent arousal of the central nervous system, which plays a part in causing the flash.

Other self-help behavioral methods include practicing self-acceptance (remind yourself, out loud if necessary, that this is a *transitory* symptom of menopause and perfectly normal), tracking the emotions and situations that precede a flash (thus putting some degree of self-control back into the equation), and trying to keep a sense of humor (share funny moments with friends who are also going through the transition).

Nagging Urogenital Signs

Vaginal dryness was the problem that prompted Penelope to try HRT. Her nurse practitioner had noticed her vaginal tissues getting thinner and drier, and this worried her. She knew that a drier vagina could eventually mean uncomfortable, even painful, sex. Another change brought on by lack of estrogen, change in the pH balance in the vagina, can lead to problems with recurrent yeast infections. One of the best ways to keep the vaginal tissues moist and thick is to use an estrogen-based cream or the insertable Estring, both of which deliver a low amount of estrogen. But the dose is enough to also lend tonicity to the base of the bladder and the urethra, which also have estrogen receptors.

In lieu of a low-dose estrogen cream, you can use Replens or Astro-Glide, two lubricants that make sexual intercourse more pleasant for women who don't lubricate as much as they did in younger years. KY Jelly is another lubricant, but some women report it's too gummy. Vaseline, or petroleum jelly, should not be used to lubricate the vagina, since it traps moisture and can help bacteria thrive.

It's most important to keep your vaginal muscles toned. That is why the prescription "use it or lose it" is applied commonly in connection with a healthy genital and urinary tract. Using your vaginal muscles can encompass masturbation as well as penile penetration. This means any sexual activity that produces an orgasm and thus contraction of the pelvic muscles. Doing Kegel exercises (see page 68) is always a good idea, both for the vagina and the bladder, and may help prevent stress incontinence, a potentially serious problem for the postmenopausal woman, in which a bit of urine is lost upon coughing, laughing, or engaging in vigorous activity.

There are many noninvasive approaches to bladder control, including limiting or eliminating caffeine, training the bladder to hold more urine, and biofeedback. If incontinence becomes a real problem, surgery may eventually be indicated. See the "Best Resources" section at the end of this chapter for sources of information on bladder and urinary incontinence problems.

Weight Gain and "The Blahs"

It's not unusual, experts say, for women to gain 5 to 10 pounds during menopause. Even if weight gain is minimal, body fat redistributes around the middle, so that women in middle age begin to

Kegel Exercises

Make these part of your daily routine. You can find the correct muscles in the pelvic floor the next time you urinate. After you have begun, simply squeeze to stop the urine stream, then release. This is the same action you must repeat several times a day to increase muscle control.

Regimens vary, but most agree that 10 repetitions two or three times a day are a good idea. Simply squeeze for a count of three seconds (count "one thousand one . . . one thousand two . . . one thousand three"), then release. You can build up to more repetitions, or to squeezing the muscles for longer periods of time. Health care practitioners agree that Kegel exercises can be an important tool in preventing problems with urinary incontinence.

Source: Janis Luft, R.N., M.S., Mt. Zion Faculty Practice, University of California at San Francisco.

resemble men in middle age. What can you do? Those 5 to 10 pounds are often more resistant to dieting than 25 or more pounds of weight were in your younger years. Weight gain can contribute to "the blahs," that state of feeling slightly down and not yourself. Overeating or drinking alcohol can then become an attempt to deal with the blahs, thus setting up a vicious cycle. Some of the tips below aimed at countering weight gain (most notably, exercise) can also address the buildup of stress.

Learn to live with the few extra pounds

Will your friends or family love you any less? Probably not. This can be an opportunity to work on some of the issues attendant to aging, such as body image (discussed in Chapter 2) and the body/ mind connection (Chapter 7).

Go on a diet

This may be harder to do during menopause, not just because of a slower metabolism, but due to the extra stressors apt to be present in your life. Look at "Readiness to Diet" criteria in Chapter 2 (page 37) to thoughtfully evaluate whether this is an option for you.

Change your eating habits

This is different from going on a diet, which often implies deprivation and hard-line goals. Health care experts recommend diets that are high in fiber, with three to five servings of fruit and vegetables every day, high in complex carbohydrates (whole grains, brown rice, pastas), and low in fatty and sugary foods.

Change your drinking habits

Red wine in moderation has been said to help prevent heart attacks, but research into breast cancer indicates that even moderate consumption (one glass of wine per day) can predispose a woman to developing breast cancer. Women handle alcohol differently from men because of a stomach enzyme that breaks down alcohol more quickly. What this means is that it takes a lot less to make women tipsy than it does men. Impaired driving ability can result, a very serious health hazard. Alcohol consumption can also lead to more falls, something that women over the age of 50 should take care to avoid because of their increased bone loss. So, take your alcohol in small amounts, less frequently, and seek help if you think you may have a problem.

Exercise

This might be the best prescription of all. In study after study, regular weight-bearing and aerobic exercise is cited for contributing to an increased sense of well-being, increased bone and muscle strength, increased stamina, and even reducing hot flashes.

If you haven't been an athletic person up until now, tackle an exercise program gradually. Both *Managing Your Menopause* and *Menopause and Midlife Health*, by Drs. Utian and Notelovitz, respectively (see "Best Resources" at the end of Chapter 1), include a series of strengthening exercises for midlife women. I recommend seeking a class with women around your age. Eventually, you'll build some camaraderie and mutual support, which, besides the immediate benefits of the exercise, will create extra inducements for continuing.

Find a menopause clinic

Finally, if you're feeling isolated and particularly troubled by a multitude of unexplainable signs and symptoms, or if you're having trouble coping with your normal routines, you may want to seek out a specialized menopause clinic. Here you'll get a full range of services, from counseling to patient education and treatments. University hospitals are a good place to start; the North American Menopause Society (see "Best Resources" at the end of Chapter 3) can also direct you to nearby clinics. Most of the treatments will probably be mainstream (that is, not alternative therapies). But this is changing as more practitioners learn how to talk with their patients about alternatives and educate themselves about which claims of complementary medicine are scientifically valid and which are not.

The next section will help you better understand the most mainstream treatment of all: hormone replacement therapy, a form of estrogen in combination with a synthetic progesterone (a progestin).

The Estrogen Question

Treatment of menopausal symptoms is the number one reason most women take HRT. Uncomfortable side effects, such as uterine bleeding and weight gain, and fear of cancer are the two reasons most women stop using HRT, and most will stop within two years of their original prescription.

Many women may be worried about making the decision of whether to start hormone replacement therapy. My first book, *Making the Estrogen Decision,* deals with the pros and cons of this decision in detail. For this section, the arguments on both sides will be summarized.

Whether to take estrogens is a serious decision, but it's not an insurmountable one. Although reasons may be urgent—for instance, early onset of osteoporosis—you often have time in which to weigh your choices. This is not like having to take antibiotics to combat pneumonia. However, I strongly urge you to do your own additional research concerning this question and to discuss with your physician and/or your nurse practitioner what you've learned. Informing yourself of common indications will be very helpful when you discuss this option with your physician. For instance, for a woman with an intact uterus, some form of progesterone, usually synthetic, is prescribed in tandem with the estrogen. This is because progesterone will guard against unchecked buildup of the uterine lining (stimulated by the estrogen to grow), and help to prevent uterine cancer.

Positive Indications for Estrogen

Estrogen is one of the most important hormonal compounds in your body. Virtually all of your body's systems are affected by its presence—your cardiovascular system, nervous system, skin, skeleton, reproductive organs and tissues, and urinary system. When your ovaries stop releasing eggs and producing estrogen, these systems are all affected—some to a greater degree than others. There are times, for instance, when estrogen replacement is a very good idea.

Premature menopause

Women who go through menopause in their late 30s or early 40s (a small but measurable group of the female population) are missing out on estrogen for a longer period of time than their peers. As a result, they may lose more bone density, or experience vaginal atrophy, or even see an increase in cholesterol levels sooner than would most women who go through a natural menopause at the average age of 50.

Surgical menopause

A complete hysterectomy in which the ovaries as well as the uterus are removed, or oophorectomy, removal of the ovaries only, are often no-debate indications for estrogen replacement. The reason is the same as for the women in premature menopause: Estrogen depletion affects many body tissues and may prematurely age women. Dosages of estrogen are typically higher for hysterectomized women because surgical removal of the ovaries brings on sudden menopause.

Uncomfortable or very noticeable symptoms during natural menopause

At the present time, the FDA-approved indications for post-menopausal estrogen are (1) atrophy of the urogenital system, (2) hot flashes, and (3) prevention of osteoporosis. (Wyeth-Ayerst, manufacturer of Premarin, the most commonly prescribed estrogen, is currently seeking FDA approval to have Premarin also listed as a preventive for cardiovascular disease because estrogen raises the level of HDL or "good" cholesterol in the blood. When estrogen is given with a progestin, however, as is required when the woman has an intact uterus, the blood cholesterol levels change in other ways and may reverse the positive cardiovascular effects of the estrogen. As mentioned earlier, the large HERS study showed no apparent benefit of HRT to women already diagnosed with heart disease. Study results are still pending from other large trials.)

Here are the common signs for which estrogens are prescribed in clinical practice:

- hot flashes
- atrophic urethritis (inflammation of the urethra)
- stress incontinence
- sensory-urge incontinence (a constant sensation of having to urinate)
- atrophic vaginitis
- dysphoric (depressed) mood
- dyspareunia (pain upon intercourse)
- decreased sexual motivation (testosterone, an androgen, may also be needed with decreased sexual desire, and you should ask your physician about this)
- prevention of chronic disease processes after menopause, specifically osteoporosis and cardiovascular disease (see Chapter 6)

Forms of Estrogen and Progesterone

Estrogens are given orally via pills, transdermally via patches and creams, and intravaginally via creams and plastic rings impregnated with estradiol that releases over a three-month period. The strength of prescriptions varies, but the standard dosage of estrogen is 0.625 mg daily. This is considered the lowest dose of estrogen effective in protecting against bone loss, although studies are now beginning to indicate there may be a benefit for a lower dose regimen (see Chapter 6, "Your Bones: Constantly Changing"). In women who have not had a hysterectomy, the estrogen is "opposed" by giving a synthetic progesterone, called a progestin, usually for a sequence of 10 to 14 days at the end of the month to induce a menstrual period. This allows any uterine lining buildup from the estrogen to slough off. Progestins are prescribed in 2.5-, 5-, and 10-mg dosages.

A variety of therapies and prescriptions are available. Some pills combine estrogen and progesterone on a daily basis, so that bleeding is nonexistent or very light. Some estrogen pills contain testosterone, a male hormone that can stimulate the libido. In the last five years alone, the number of pharmaceutical products for hormone replacement has increased exponentially. In the summer of 1999, a physician could prescribe any one of six oral estrogen tablets (Estrace, EstraTab, Menest, Ogen, Ortho-Est, and the most popular, Premarin); five estrogen transdermal patches (Alora, Climara, Estraderm, FemPatch, and Vivelle); four estrogen vaginal creams (Estrace, Ogen, Ortho, and Premarin); or one vaginal ring (Estring). Progestins are available in oral form (Amen, Aygestin, Cycrin, Megace, Micronor, Prometrium, and Provera) and as an intravaginal gel (Crinone gel). Then there is the breakthrough combination of the two hormones—CombiPatch or Premphase plus Prempro, the two latter being oral tablets. Table 4-1 gives a sampling of the variety of prescription medications.

Keep in mind that estrogens are primarily given to alleviate hot flashes, relieve vaginal dryness and urinary complaints, and promote denser bones. Progesterone also relieves hot flashes, but is mainly given to oppose the estrogen (that is, to provide a counterbalance against estrogen's stimulation of the uterine lining to

Table 4-1   Estrogens and Progestins Used for Hormone Therapy

Brand Name	Generic Name	Manufacturer
Estrogens		
Oral		
Cenestin	Synthetic conjugated estrogens	Duramed Pharmaceuticals
Estrace	Micronized estradiol	Mead Johnson Laboratories
EstraTab	Esterified estrogen	Solvay Pharmaceuticals
Menest	Esterified estrogen	Monarch Pharmaceuticals
Ogen	Estropipate	Upjohn
Ortho-Est	Estropipate	Ortho Pharmaceuticals
Premarin	Conjugated equine estrogens	Ayerst Labs
Transdermal Patches		
Alora	Estradiol	Procter & Gamble
Climara	Estradiol	Berlex
Estraderm	Estradiol	Novartis
FemPatch	Estradiol	Parke-Davis
Vivelle	Estradiol	Ciba-Geigy
Vaginal Creams		
Estrace	Estradiol	Mead Johnson Laboratories
Ogen	Estropipate	Upjohn
Ortho	Dinestrol	Ortho Pharmaceuticals
Premarin	Conjugated equine estrogens	Ayerst Labs
Vaginal Ring		
Estring	Estradiol	Pharmacia & Upjohn
Progestins		
Oral		
Amen	Medroxyprogesterone acetate	Carnick Laboratories
Aygestin	Norethindrone acetate	ESI-Lederle
Cycrin	Medroxyprogesterone acetate	ESI-Lederle
Megace	Megestrol acetate	Mead Johnson
Micronor	Norethindrone acetate	Ortho-McNeil
Prometrium	Micronized progesterone	Solvay Pharmaceuticals
Provera	Medroxyprogesterone acetate	Upjohn

Table 4-1 *continued*

Intravaginal

Crinone gel   Progesterone   Ayerst Labs

Estrogen/Progestin Combinations

CombiPatch   Estradiol/Norethindrone acetate   Rhone-Poulenc

Premphase (oral)   Conjugated equine estrogens/   Wyeth-Ayerst
                     Medroxyprogesterone acetate

Prempro (oral)   Conjugated equine estrogens/   Wyeth-Ayerst
                     Medroxyprogesterone acetate

Sources: Office of Technology Assessment, 1992. *Physicians' Desk Reference*; Solvay Pharmaceuticals; Wyeth-Ayerst; Chuck Adams, Pharm.D., Rite-Aid Pharmacies, 1999.

grow, which can lead to precancerous conditions). Side effects of estrogens can include bleeding and spotting, bloating, breast tenderness, headache, and nausea. Except for nausea, these same side effects are also possible with progesterones, although there is a higher likelihood of mood swings with a progestin.

Other Sources of Hormones

Some women want more natural sources of hormones than they get at the standard pharmacy. They may be sensitive to the effects of synthetic estradiol, conjugated equine estrogens, or synthetic progestins. Suffering with hot flashes or diagnosed with bone loss, they may seek hormone replacement in more "natural" forms. One estrogen preparation getting a lot of recent attention is Tri-Est, a mixture of estrone, estradiol, and estriol, in a 1:1:8 ratio. Because estriol is a weaker estrogen, many claim that it may reduce the risk of developing breast cancer. However, there is no solid evidence to date, according to Adriane Fugh-Berman, M.D., writing in *Alternative Therapies in Women's Health*, that Tri-Est is safe for the endometrium or breast tissue.

Natural progesterone, derived from the Mexican wild yam, is also touted as a remedy for a large range of conditions, from PMS to protecting bone. Again, the evidence is not yet in. However, many physicians are now writing prescriptions for micronized natural progesterones, which come in a powder form and must be formulated by a compounding pharmacy. In dosages ranging from 25 to 300 mg, it can take the form of an oral capsule, a lozenge dissolved under the tongue, or vaginal or rectal suppositories. Many small pharmacies now make compounds to order with a prescription. If this service is not available at your local pharmacy, see the "Best Resources" list of organizations for the Women's International Pharmacy, which will ship anywhere in the United States.

Reasons Not to Take Estrogens

As with the positive indications for taking estrogen, the reasons *not* to take estrogen include many gray areas. There are some absolute contraindications, some currently under debate, and others that may be a matter of individual choice. These are described in Table 4-2.

Although it might seem as if the reasons *not* to take estrogen outweigh the reasons to take it, what is most important about this process is that you be aware of your own benefit-to-risk ratio. Does early heart disease (heart attack before age 55) or high cholesterol run in your family? Did your grandmother have a crippling dowager's hump (a sign of osteoporosis)? Do you have endometriosis? Compile a list with pros on one side, cons on the other, and picture a balance scale. Remember that some factors will get more weight than others. For instance, a family history of heart disease might outweigh your natural resistance to taking pills every day.

Take time to weigh your decision carefully. If, after looking at the balance sheet, you decide hormone replacement is definitely not for you, you may want to take a noninvasive health care course. By that, I mean using good, practical common sense. And remember your yearly checkups—a good idea at any age. According to nurse practitioner Margaret King, R.N., of San Luis Obispo, California, a woman must be prepared to put more energy into self-care if she is not going to take hormone replacement. If you decide that HRT would have positive benefits for you, be prepared to deal with some side effects. Most reproductive endocrinologists agree that a therapy should be adhered to for at

The Physical Effects of Menopause: Managing Your Symptoms ∞ 77

Table 4-2   Reasons Not to Take Estrogens

Absolutely Not	Under Debate	Perhaps Not
Undiagnosed uterine bleeding		Uterine leiomyoma (fibroids)
Suspected breast cancer	History of breast cancer	
Suspected endometrial cancer	History of endometrial cancer	Endometriosis
Active venous thrombosis*		History of pregnancy-related thrombosis*
		History of oral contraceptive-related thrombosis*
	Malignant melanoma	

Other conditions to be discussed and evaluated with physician

		History of cholelithiasis (gallstones)
		History of migraine
		Hypertriglyceridemia (excess triglycerides in the blood)
		Liver disease

*Tendency for blood clots to form.

Source: Gail A. Greendale, M.D., and Howard L. Judd, M.D., "The Menopause: Health Implications and Clinical Management," *Journal of the American Geriatrics Society*, 41:4 (April 1993), p. 433.

least three months before deciding it's not working or that the side effects are not bearable. Keep track of any side effects, such as unexpected bleeding or dizziness, and report them to your doctor.

Before and During HRT

Because noncontraceptive estrogen and progestin will have effects on your body's systems, it's imperative that you be monitored for possible changes in the endometrium, blood cholesterol, and

An example of a possible "yes" to HRT might look like this:

Reasons For	Reasons Against
Disruptive hot flashes	History of migraine*
Vaginal atrophy	
Family heart disease	
Early menopause	
Serious bone loss from steroid use	

*Note: A history of migraine would warrant monitoring your progress with HRT closely.

A probable "no" to HRT might look like this:

Reasons For	Reasons Against
Hot flashes	Sister with breast cancer
Drying vagina	Undiagnosed vaginal bleeding

This woman might want to try other remedies for her hot flashes, and non-hormonal lubricants for her vaginal symptoms. And, obviously, she and her doctor should be pursuing a diagnosis for her vaginal bleeding.

other factors. Most researchers agree that it generally takes three months on the therapy to see whether it is yielding the proper results. If you start to get breakthrough bleeding on a continuous regimen of estrogen and progestin daily, you should consult your physician. Course corrections should be tried if the first, second, or even third regimen does not work for you. Taking estrogen and progestin in a cyclic manner can convert the bleeding to a scheduled period each month. Or a lower dose of estrogen may stimulate the uterine lining less, thus reducing the bleeding. Consult "Your Before and During HRT Checklist."

Your Before and During HRT Checklist

Regular Screenings Before HRT

Pelvic exam

Urinalysis

Blood pressure check

Fasting blood sugars

Cholesterol levels, including HDL, LDL, and triglycerides

Liver function test

Thyroid function

Pap smear

Mammogram

Regular Screenings While on HRT

Annual Pap smear

Annual mammogram, if over 50

Pelvic and rectal exam

Semiannual tests: blood pressure, red blood cell count, clinical breast exam, urinalysis

Monthly breast self-examination

Alternative Approaches

Many women in menopause feel that traditional Western medicine does not offer them enough alternatives, and they therefore seek out other healing methods to deal with their symptoms. Practitioners of alternative healing methods—acupuncturists, homeopaths, herbalists—view menopause quite differently from most Western practitioners. In Chinese medicine, for instance, menopause signals the beginning of a woman's real life, the time when she begins to attain wisdom. Perhaps it is this view that makes alternative medicine seem so refreshing to Westerners who have grown up with a popular culture that worships youth. In addition, the Eastern approach takes the mind and emotions into consideration when addressing a person's overall health.

What constitutes an alternative approach? To some strictly mainstream physicians, chiropractors are considered alternative practitioners. To others, alternative approaches might mean following a strict vegetarian diet and engaging in daily meditation. The term is relative, and that is part of the problem. In this country, alternative practitioners are usually not licensed and not bound by the same standards as those in the mainstream medical profession. Add to this the difference in underlying philosophies, and you're often comparing apples and walnuts when you contrast Western with Eastern therapeutic approaches. What follows are short capsule descriptions of various alternative therapies relevant to menopausal women.

Chinese Medicine/Acupuncture

In Chinese medicine, the body is seen as an integrated system of 14 energy channels called meridians, which are associated with various organs. If energy becomes blocked along any of these meridians, it can trigger imbalance in the body, leading to the disease process. In menopausal women, imbalance in the kidneys can lead to too much hot energy and too little water energy, inducing frequent hot flashes. Ways to treat these imbalances include acupuncture and herbal remedies.

Acupuncture may also be helpful to relieve aches and pains associated with menopause, such as arthralgia (pain in the joints) and myalgia (generalized muscle pains). The procedure involves insertion of fine, long needles into one of the body's 361 acupuncture points to release the flow of energy. Although recorded and anecdotal evidence reveals that acupuncture works, we still do not understand why it can be an effective tool for chronic pain and arthritis and can be used in lieu of anesthesia during surgical procedures. A 1989 University of California, Irvine, study documented Chinese patients undergoing surgery. Their pain was blocked, but the scientists could not explain how, except to sug-

Finding a Good Acupuncturist

- Licensing: A current license must be displayed. For instance, in California, acupuncturists must be licensed by the:

   Acupuncture Committee
   1420 Howe Ave., Suite 14
   Sacramento, CA 95825

   Check with your state's board of quality assurance regarding acupuncturists.

- Cleanliness, safety: Check out the office. Is it clean? Are the linens or paper linings on the examining tables changed after each patient? Are disposable or autoclave-sterilized needles used?

gest that acupuncture blocked the perception of pain—perhaps the needles somehow release endorphins, natural opiates produced by the body. Whatever its mechanism of action, acupuncture does seem to work for some people.

Susan Lange, an acupuncturist and practitioner formerly with the Meridian Center in Santa Monica, California, explains that a woman's hot flashes are indicative of an imbalance with the kidneys, an imbalance related to the coolness of water. Acupuncture treatments focusing on the kidney meridian can revive that water energy, thus bringing the hot element (hot flashes) into control. "Acupuncture," she notes, "is very much a way of regulating the body, strengthening the parts that are weaker and balancing those out with the parts that are too strong."

While these methods may work, no clinical and long-term studies have investigated why or how. My advice is to seek out an acupuncturist who is licensed by a state board and to avoid anyone who makes promises of an absolute cure or of restoring you to perfect health.

Chiropractic

Chiropractors treat physical injuries with a combination of techniques, most of them related to physical therapy: massage, ultrasound massage, and spinal manipulation. Since joint and muscle pain are often part of the complex of menopausal symptoms, women may seek relief from a chiropractor or masseuse. Use the accompanying tips for finding a reputable chiropractor.

Homeopathy

Founded by Samuel Hahnemann in the 18th century, this system of therapeutics treats diseases based on the "law of similars": Like cures like. To treat sick people, remedies are used that are capable of producing toxic effects in healthy people. These oral remedies, given in minute doses as a tincture or solution, alleviate the same symptoms they cause in large doses by stimulating the body's natural defense system. There are over 400 homeopathic remedies, including arsenic, sulfur, and ipecac. Most homeopaths who practice have licenses and most do lengthy case histories when they first see patients.

Herbal Remedies/Naturopaths

"The eclectics" is a term I use for those who blend theories from various disciplines, prescribe herbal remedies, and even participate with mainstream practitioners in treating menopausal women. They offer a plethora of natural remedies for hot flashes, insomnia, anxiety attacks, and other physical and emotional complaints of the climacteric. Janet Zand, a well-known acupuncturist, homeopath, and doctor of oriental medicine in southern California, advises her clients to pay attention to all aspects of self-care. Her advice to midlife women includes:

- Establish an exercise routine. "It's probably our most powerful antiaging device," she says. "You could have created the perfect diet for yourself, taking the perfect supplements, perfect herbs, but if you're not exercising, that perfect nutritional information doesn't get to circulate throughout your body. I

Finding a Reliable Chiropractor

- Call the American Chiropractic Association in Arlington, Virginia, at (703) 276-8800 to obtain referrals to a chiropractor in your state; or call your state chiropractic association.

- When you call or first visit the office, ask about licensing and accreditation. The doctor should hold a degree from a reputable college. Any additional training should also be through an accredited association. Beware of someone who holds a "Diplomate of Spinology," for instance, which may have come from an unaccredited source.

- Be able to recognize a sales pitch. Are you being fit into a program rather than being treated as an individual? Does the doctor spend a lot of money on advertising? While this is not an immediate disqualifier, it does give you clues that perhaps the practitioner is more into marketing than further education in treating patients.

- Does the chiropractor maintain you'll have to keep coming indefinitely? The doctor should be able to give you a range of weeks or months within which your condition can be resolved.

- Question the doctor about his or her referral patterns. If a diagnosis is outside his or her area of expertise, will you be referred to neurologists or orthopedists? A reputable chiropractor will most likely have referral rela-

think exercise enhances the functioning of the entire endocrine system and, of course, the metabolism."

- Eating tips: Gradually decrease saturated fat, increase fiber, limit alcohol consumption, eat dietary sources of calcium that agree with you (especially the dark green leafy vegetables), and keep caffeine "to a low roar."

Table 4-3   Some Herbs Used for Menopause Symptoms
(Read labels for recommended dosages.)

Herb	Used For
Bupleurum or Ch'ai Hu	Clearing the liver; in combination with dong quai to reduce anxiety
Dong quai	Alleviating PMS and menstrual cramps; in combination with bupleurum and peony root to combat anxiety, depression, insomnia, and hot flashes
Peony root	Relaxing the nervous system
Milk thistle	Protecting the liver; used as an adjunct with HRT
Vitex or chaste tree	Stimulating pituitary; alleviating PMS and discomforts of menopause
Red raspberry leaf	Replacing folic acid lost during menopause; toning the uterus
Skullcap	Tranquilizing and sedating effects
Valerian	Sedating effects
Passion flower	Calming effects
Oat straw	Calming properties; improving absorption of calcium
Chamomile	Soothing and calming effects
St. John's wort	Relieving anxiety
Siberian ginseng	Alleviating hot flashes, insomnia, and agitated depression; regulating blood sugar
American ginseng	Alleviating perimenopausal fatigue and exhaustion

Zand prescribes a whole range of herbs for clients' menopausal symptoms. (See Table 4-3.) She admits that one of the problems with herbal remedies for the public at large is the lack of scientific study. Often clients come to her who cannot take HRT (because of breast cancer or other risk factors) and yet want to deal with their menopausal symptoms. Her advice to women who are not near urban areas, where herbalists are more likely to practice, is to choose one or two herbs from Table 4-3 or a combination blend found in health food stores and start "very gingerly, very slowly. Maybe in the beginning you just take an herb three times a week, then increase to every day. The next week you use other herbs, always alternating what you are using."

"Herbs are just food," she notes, "but they happen to be concentrated food. If you treat them as such and know that you're not going to eat one every single day and you rotate, you are going to do very well." Just as the seasons change, so will your use of herbs. In the winter, "you're going to need more strong, rooty-type herbs, just as we tend to eat more rooty-type vegetables and heavier food in the winter. In the summer, we eat lighter, more leafy foods. It's the same with herbs."

Herbal remedies can be quite helpful, but again, don't forget to question solutions to health problems that you read or hear about. For instance, Rosemary Gladstar, founder of the Traditional Medicinals Tea Company and the California School of Herbal Studies, recommends in a *Prevention* magazine article, "for osteoporosis pain, try salves that have penetrating essential oils such as sage, rosemary, camphor, eucalyptus, and peppermint. You can use Tiger Balm or even Vick's VapoRub, which contains camphor, eucalyptus and menthol." If a woman actually has *pain* from osteoporosis, she should be under a doctor's care, preferably an orthopedist, endocrinologist, or both. Pain from osteoporosis could mean a very serious condition with porous bones, and she needs to find a way to stabilize her already fragile skeleton. Any amount of penetrating salve is not going to get at the root problem.

Is Soy the Answer?

Some women I've interviewed swear by soy milk and tofu as powerful antidotes to hot flashes. Soy products contain isoflavones, also known as phytoestrogens (plant estrogens), and they have a mild estrogenlike effect. It is also thought that soy products can prevent breast cancer, but this is a conclusion based on epidemiological evidence (studies of large populations) demonstrating that Japanese women, who eat larger amounts of soy, get less breast cancer than their Western counterparts. Currently, at the National Center for Complementary and Alternative Medicine, there are several ongoing trials to compare soy to placebo to see whether soy is actually effective against menopausal symptoms. As far as protection against bone loss, the amount of estrogens derived from this plant source is too low a dosage to make much difference.

Dr. Robert Lindsay, president of the National Osteoporosis Foundation, has concerns about the use of phytoestrogens. Their use is very prevalent in menopausal women. "What I find disturbing is that even in women who are taking standard hormone replacement therapy, more than one-third are also taking phytoestrogens. There is very little outcome-driven data with those sorts of products," he cautioned. "We know little about the effects by themselves, but we know absolutely nothing about what the effects may be when taking them in combination with standard hormone replacement therapy. I think that it's potentially dangerous."

Making Sense of It All

It can be a mistake to rely wholly on "natural" remedies for serious health problems. Be wary of any generalized promises, such as that you will be led to "perfect health." Even alternative practitioners such as homeopaths agree that health is an ongoing process, and the body is constantly in a state of flux.

Approach these types of practitioners with a healthy dose of "confident skepticism," as Janine O'Leary Cobb advises. We often complain that Western medicine undertakes insufficient research to warn us of dangerous side effects. Similarly, it helps to remember that all sorts of "alternative" methods exist for which there is no "proof" from any empirical testing that the method is safe and/or effective. "Even the published studies from Europe," points out Dr. Paul Stumpf, "are often not the type of research that we are accustomed to evaluating in the United States. For example, trials may not include a placebo; they may be comparing alternative therapies to each other. Or they may rely largely on anecdotal evidence and it's very difficult to get a handle on that."

Dr. John Renner, former president of the National Council for Reliable Health Information, put it more bluntly: Taking remedies that have not been scientifically validated is like "trying to navigate with a flat earth map!" Consumers can only be truly empowered if they are making decisions based on empirical evidence. The checklist on page 87 for spotting an unproved remedy can be of help, and several other resources are listed at the end of this chapter.

Checklist for Spotting an Unproven Remedy

Is It Likely to Work for Me?

Suspect an unproven remedy if it:

- Claims to work for all types of menopausal as well as other health problems.
- Uses only case histories or testimonials as proof.
- Cites only one study as proof. (A single study only suggests that a treatment may have promise. Usually, a number of scientists must repeat the same study and get similar results to prove that the treatment works.)
- Cites a study without a control group. (In clinical trials, one group of people, the experimental group, gets a new treatment. Another group, the control group, gets either no treatment or one whose effects are already known. These comparisons help show that the results of the study are attributable to the new treatment and not to some other factor.)

How Safe Is It?

Suspect an unproven remedy if it:

- Comes without any directions for proper use.
- Does not list contents.
- Has no information or warnings about side effects.
- Is described as harmless or natural.

How Is It Promoted?

Suspect an unproven remedy if it:

- Claims it's based on a secret formula.
- Claims it cures all menopausal symptoms.
- Is available only from one source.
- Is promoted only in the media, in books, or by mail order.

Source: Adapted from "Arthritis Unproven Remedies," Arthritis Foundation, © 1987; used by permission.

In the next chapter, I'll discuss the challenges of sexuality in the years beyond menopause and how you can best prepare to meet them.

Best Resources

Books

Natural Menopause, The Complete Guide to a Woman's Most Misunderstood Passage, by Susan Perry and Katherine O'Hanlan, M.D. Perseus, 1996; 208 pages; $15.00.

A commonsense, well-rounded book, written in friendly and accessible language. Dr. O'Hanlan and Ms. Perry cover "The Great Hormone Debate," sexuality after menopause, and "taking charge" with proper exercise, nutrition, and skin care.

Making the Estrogen Decision, by Gretchen Henkel. Lowell House, Los Angeles, 1992; 221 pages; $21.95.

An in-depth look at the pros and cons of hormone replacement therapy, featuring interviews with physicians, researchers, and women wrestling with the estrogen decision. Emphasizes information gathering and empowers the reader to make the decision that is right for her.

What Women Should Know About Menopause, by Judith Sachs. Dell Medical Library, New York, 1991; paperback, 149 pages; $3.99.

Sensible, straightforward, and succinct, this is one of the best books on menopause, written by a woman whose other medical titles include *What Women Can Do About Chronic Endometriosis* (also by Dell Medical Library). Ms. Sachs covers the territory well, and includes some information on alternative therapies, in balanced fashion.

Alternative Books

The Alternative Medicine Handbook, by Barrie R. Cassileth, Ph.D. Norton, New York, 1999; paperback, 340 pages; $19.95.

Alternative Medicine: What Works: A Comprehensive, Easy-to-Read Review of the Scientific Evidence, Pro and Con, by Adriane Fugh-Berman, M.D. Williams & Wilkins, Philadelphia, 1997; paperback, 254 pages; $17.95.

Dr. Fugh-Berman works for the National Institutes of Health, is highly respected, and brings a measured perspective to the alternative medicine debate.

Earl Mindell's New Herb Bible, by Earl Mindell, R.Ph., Ph.D. Fireside Books, Simon and Schuster, New York, 2000; paperback, 320 pages; $14.00.

A compendium of commonly used herbs, their uses, proper dosages, and cautions about overdosing. Written in a friendly style, informative about the history of herbal medicine.

Fundamentals of Complementary and Alternative Medicine, 2d ed., by Marc S. Micozzi, M.D., and C. Everett Koop, M.D. Mosby-Year-Book, St. Louis, 2001; paperback, 430 pages; $49.00.

Another measured look at complementary and alternative medicine by the esteemed Dr. Koop and coauthor Dr. Micozzi.

Organizations

American Chiropractic Association
1701 Clarendon Boulevard, 2d Floor
Arlington, VA 22209
(703) 276-8800
www.amerchiro.org

Call the association for a referral to a chiropractor in your state, or for the number of your state's local chiropractic association.

American Massage Therapy Association (AMTA)
820 Davis Street, Suite 100
Evanston, IL 60201-4444
(847) 864-0123
www.amtamassage.org

Call AMTA's association office for referrals to members in your area. The association's 29,000 members work in different modalities of massage therapy, including Swedish massage, acupressure, reflexology, and aroma therapy.

American Association of Naturopathic Physicians
8201 Greensboro Drive, Suite 300
McLean, VA 22101
(703) 610-9037
www.naturopathic.org

Click on "Public Entrance" to find definitions of what a naturopathic doctor (N.D.) does and to access a database of association members by geographic area. While most do not specialize in as specific an area as menopausal helath, many hold additional certifications in acupuncture, herbal medicine, and acupressure. Naturopathic physicians in most states must work under the supervision of an M.D., but 10 states allow naturopaths to diagnose and treat patients on their own.

The National Council Against Health Fraud
www.ncahf.org

Maintained by Webmaster Stephen Barrett, M.D., this agency was the brainchild of Dr. John Renner, cited in this book and now deceased. The private, nonprofit agency focuses on health misinformation, fraud, and quackery as public health problems. NCAHF furnishes position papers on acupncture, chiropractic, and herbal remedies, as well as links to other sites, such as "Quackwatch."

National Kidney and Urologic Diseases
Information Clearinghouse
3 Information Way
Bethesda, MD 20892-3580
(800) 891-5388
www.niddk.nih.gov

Established in 1987, the clearinghouse provides information about diseases of the kidneys and urologic system to the public and health care professionals. A section called "Menopause and Bladder Control" on the clearinghouse Web site gives basic overview information and provides links to other resources.

National Women's Health Network
514 10th Street N.W., Suite 400
Washington, DC 20004
(202) 347-1140
www.womenshealthnetwork.org

A women's health care advocacy group, National Women's Health Network provides information and position papers on many aspects of women's health, from abortion to fibroids, from hysterectomy to PMS. You can get a complete list of titles by calling the organization. One booklet in particular, "Taking Hormones and Women's Health," may be helpful in rounding out your research on HRT. The booklet can be obtained by contacting the network.

Women's International Pharmacy
5708 Monona Drive
Madison, WI 53716
(608) 221-7800
(800) 279-5708

Also,

13925 W. Meeker Boulevard, Suite 13
Sun City West, AZ 85375
(800) 279-5708
www.womensinternational.com

This organization, like many other compounding pharmacies, makes prescriptions to order for physicians and also sells directly to consumers. Compounds, such as natural progesterone from natural ingredients, can be made to order with a doctor's prescription. An information packet is available free of charge by calling the 800 number, and knowledgeable pharmacists are available to answer customers' questions.

CHAPTER FIVE

Sex During and After Menopause

> Is part of menopause being turned off? Is that supposed to be part of it?
>
> *Participant in a radio show entitled "My Dinner with Menopause," produced for "Soundprint" and aired on National Public Radio*

In many ways, issues about sex and sexuality are at the center of our anxieties about menopause. In our culture, being sexually active means that one is vital, young, a "player" in the game. Both men and women are subjected to narrow definitions of vitality, but at menopause women may be especially conscious of cultural stereotypes. If a woman loses self-esteem because she sees her attractiveness waning, it can affect her sexual activity as much as physical causes.

In our media- and advertising-saturated culture, youth and thinness are synonymous with desirability. Although we're constantly bombarded with all sorts of sexual images used to sell everything from beer to deodorant, personal expression of sexuality still remains a very private thing. We've all become modern and sophisticated in the level at which we're capable of talking about the problems of sex. But even for the most worldly of women, talking about the practical details and mechanics of sex, even with friends, can be uncomfortable.

Sometimes broaching the subject with your partner can be awkward—perhaps more so than with friends. If your sexual responses are changing, as they are likely to do during menopause, this clearly affects your partner as well. Some women report that when sex became painful because of a dry vagina, they and their partners became reticent to initiate sexual contact. You both may be feeling vulnerable at this particular time. As the changes of menopause (weight gain, less vaginal lubrication) begin to take place, you may also feel less desirable, and thus more insecure about your sexuality. Adjusting to so many losses can easily become overwhelming. It's important not to let insecurity isolate you; one of the best antidotes is communication. And with so much attention being focused on menopause, you're not alone in bringing up the subject of sex during middle age.

Of course, we deal with sex during our entire lives. The various issues surrounding sexuality are omnipresent across the continuum of life's ages, according to psychotherapist and sex therapist Wendy Schain, Ph.D., of Long Beach Memorial Hospital. Such issues, however, receive special attention during menopause. So many dramatic physiologic changes (for example, hot flashes) occur concurrently with sexual changes (for example, vaginal dryness) that we can use these signs, says Schain, as a legitimate basis for discussing sexuality. Being able to use medical issues for broaching discussion about sex comes almost as a relief, especially in our American culture, where often, paradoxically, repressed attitudes and excessive openness about sex coexist. The bottom line, says Schain, is that "we all get a lot more comfortable" talking about sex.

"The reality of menopause is that the target areas for the physiologic changes are the sex organs," she says. "It is a little hard to deny this. And it allows us to say, 'Okay, we can talk about this topic more comfortably and not have to apologize or be embarrassed about it.'" A quick glance at the women's health section in bookstores (or a daytime tour of talk shows) attests to the new candor about our libidos.

Now that everyone's talking about sexuality and menopause, how are sexual concerns being handled? In the professional arena, researchers continue to study and analyze human sexual response, and to educate their colleagues through articles, forums, and conferences about proper approaches to the menopausal woman with sexual complaints. Whereas family practitioners and some gynecologists might have once routinely referred a woman with loss of libido to a psychiatrist, they may now be more likely to first investigate hormonal causes.

In the studies that have measured sexual difficulties in menopausal women, a majority of women report at least some modification in sexual functioning during the climacteric. The changes cover a range of problems from lack of desire to less frequent intercourse to painful intercourse. Medical literature is now filled with articles by experts studying and treating sexual dysfunction who urge their colleagues to undertake adequate medical histories and hormone level testing and to educate their patients about the scope of menopausal symptoms.

In addition to physicians' willingness to acknowledge the physiological basis for sexual difficulties, the other bit of good news is that increasing numbers of practitioners, both traditional and alternative, are taking into account both the emotional and physical aspects of their patients; that is, they're finally beginning to treat the whole person. Nowhere does this make as much sense as in the area of sexuality. Because human sexual response is a phenomenon of interdependent factors, sexual problems are best seen in a multidisciplinary context, using an interweaving of biological, societal, psychological, and cultural models.

Eastern medicine sees sexuality as an expression of the body's balance or imbalance. A woman's loss of desire for sex may be an indication that energies in one or more of her vital organs are either blocked or "out-expressing" the other organs. For instance, a woman who loves her partner but doesn't desire sex may have too much "heart" energy. Diagnosis and treatment, in this instance making use of acupuncture or herbal remedies (see Chapter 4), would help to tone down the heart energy, allowing her sexual energies to emerge.

Western disciplines may take a two-pronged approach. Some attribute loss of libido to a hormonal imbalance, while other practitioners might look for a psychological component. The cause can be either, or both. In this chapter, you'll learn about various approaches to sexual problems and lack of desire, and how to find your way to the right solutions as well as how to dispel outdated notions.

Does Menopause Spell the End of Desire?

Like the woman in the beginning of this chapter, many of us want to know: How will menopause affect my sex life? Although a host of myths about a woman's middle years and beyond have been dispelled, many still fear that menopause means the end of sex. You will more than likely experience changes, but by being aware of the reasons for them and being able to ask for treatment, you stand a greater chance of enjoying your sexuality. Although the transitional years can be upsetting, something quite wonderful appears to happen after the passage: Women begin to feel more comfortable with themselves. And, feeling more whole, they're more apt to allow themselves to feel enjoyment.

The Range of Experience

Poet/healer Deena Metzger, 57, relates some of her experiences with growing older:

> *I still experience this other self which is actually this part of me that's about 35. I really mean this—in terms of my energy, my enthusiasm. On a recent visit to the UCLA campus, as I walked around I looked at all these young men coming toward me. And it didn't occur to me that I wasn't their age and that they weren't looking at me in terms of being an attractive woman. And I felt all of that sexual buzz. . . . So it's like there are those two parts and my life is not tamed, in any way.*

Jane O'Reilly, writing in *Choices for Retirement Living* (March 1993), reports that she revels in her now invisible state:

> *I don't exactly know what happened to me. One day I was glamorous, and then, after about five years of transitional depression, I was free. They were not the best five years of my life (although they weren't the worst). My thermostat went haywire, life seemed entirely pointless, I gained 80 pounds, and I became, despite my bulk, invisible to men.*

While some women may recoil in horror at the prospect of becoming fat and asexual after menopause, O'Reilly sees her gain as freedom from the tyranny of always having to be sexy and beautiful: "I don't have to cultivate anyone or worry about making connections."

Of course, as with almost every other phase of menopause, you'll experience these changes in your own individual way. There may be days when you don't feel at peace with advancing age and can't face looking at all the new wrinkles, or skin that's becoming paper-thin, "like crushed silk," as Metzger describes it.

A lot will depend on the kinds and intensity of menopausal symptoms you have. Even more important, if you are prepared and have the right kind of support from your partner, friends, and health care practitioners, this transition need not be traumatic for your sex life. "It appears that delineation of etiologic [causative] factors and professional help can make a major difference in adjusting to menopausal changes and in maintaining a satisfying sex life," states Philip M. Sarrel, M.D., of Yale School of Medicine and a top researcher in this field, writing in the journal *Obstetrics and Gynecology Clinics of North America.*

You might, in fact, experience a new burst of sexual expression. Take Jane, age 50, who comments below on how the beginning of menopause is affecting her feelings about sex.

> I never *feel like menopause impedes my sex life! I'm very fortunate that I have a man who is not losing interest. Now sometimes he jokes, because of my hot flashes and things, that the next woman he marries isn't going to be under 70. But I always joke back that the next man I marry will be under 70! He's been really very good about trying to make concessions to me over the fact that I'm having these bodily changes.*
>
> *And I enjoy sex even more, because of my being comfortable with myself. I can enjoy it more and focus less on my—how can I say it?—my vanity. I find that the older I get, the more able I am to enjoy myself without having to be caught up in the side things about sexuality—especially things like, "How do I look? Is my stomach too fat today?"*
>
> *I think sex is one of the great joys in life, one of the great pleasures, like eating wonderful food and seeing beautiful art. I'm a very sensual person. I love all the beauty of life around me and this is one more beautiful thing. It's the most*

*intimate expression of love, but it's different things at differ-
ent times. It's not always the same thing—sometimes it's
funny, even! I love the fact that I have a man who loves it
that much, that I still feel desired and I still have those
feelings.*

Her son raised and married, her entrepreneurial business well
established, and her second marriage now in its fifth year, Jane's
in a good position to enjoy the newfound freedom of no birth
control, no periods, and no young children underfoot—except
for a beloved granddaughter who comes to visit. The open communication she and her husband enjoy adds much to their sexual
enjoyment.

What Studies Reveal

According to studies concerning the sexual satisfaction of midlife
men and women conducted by Sonya and John McKinlay of the
New England Research Institute in Watertown, Massachusetts,
menopause doesn't necessarily cause a great upheaval in our sexual
lives. There is ample anecdotal evidence of this reported by
women and therapists alike. Mary, a woman of 60, explains, "You
can do anything you want. As often as you want. It does not affect
your sexual drive at all. I haven't found anything yet that does."
Karen Lee Fontaine, professor of nursing at Purdue University
Calumet and certified sex therapist, notes that "for the women
who are really working on finding out who they are and where
they're going, there's really something nice about the age of 50."
Women who enjoy sex at this age attribute their enjoyment in part
to their growing sense of wholeness.

But other researchers, from Kinsey in the 1950s to Masters
and Johnson in the 1960s to Pfeiffer and colleagues in the 1970s,
have reported a dramatically different story. Depending on the
study, anywhere from 31 to 48 percent of American women experience a decline in sexual response and activity during and after
menopause. Likewise, Swedish and Swiss studies have reported decreased frequency and satisfaction during sex. And confounding
most of our perceptions that other cultures have fewer problems

with the transition, a survey by Philip Sarrel and colleagues of postmenopausal Nigerian women in Lagos found many of the same complaints about dyspareunia (painful intercourse) and decreased sexual activity. In fact, by nine years postmenopause, nearly 70 percent of the Nigerian women were sexually inactive. (Many opposite examples are found in other cultures, however, where older women actually gain stature and sexual partners after menopause.) Then, too, it may be that these studies, most of which are conducted through menopause clinics, where women come because of menopausal complaints, are attracting a disproportionate number of women who have difficulties during menopause.

The Physiology of Sexual Changes

You already know that when estrogen levels decrease, a woman's vaginal tissues become thinner. She also experiences a diminished amount of vaginal lubrication when sexually aroused. These two conditions can lead to pain with penetration (dyspareunia) and secondarily to involuntary and painful muscle spasms of the vagina (vaginismus), which can impede penetration.

Besides making sex uncomfortable or even painful, vaginal dryness can cause other difficulties. A woman who's never had problems with yeast infections may suddenly develop them. Couple this with bladder conditions that may also occur due to lack of estrogen, and sex may be the furthest thing from her mind!

As for the physiological reasons for lowered libido or sex drive, sexual desire is a complex set of psychological and endocrine-facilitated mechanisms, with both estrogens and testosterone (an androgen also produced in the ovaries) playing a role. While short-term estrogen therapy can improve psychological symptoms, maintain vaginal lubrication, decrease vaginal atrophy, and increase pelvic blood flow, there are other women, according to Sarrel, who require more than estrogen alone to improve psychological dysfunction, decreased sexual desire, or other sexual problems associated with menopause. Clinical studies have shown, he points out, that HRT with estrogen plus androgens provides greater improvement in symptoms such as lack of concentration, depression, fatigue, and sexual symptoms than does estrogen alone. This has been found in women who have had a surgical menopause or a natural one.

Other Physical Changes

Even for those whose sexual concerns are relatively minor, the physical changes brought on by declining estrogens in the body can present many challenges. "Penetration is really a problem," complains Helen, who's now 59. "I'm on HRT, but I didn't start it until a year ago, so I'm not sure if it's helping me or not. Also, because I'm taking the combined hormones, I find I'm having really heavy periods and cramping. That doesn't exactly help me feel in a sexy mood!"

Not only are the cells lining the vagina affected by estrogen loss, the vaginal muscles can also lose their tone. While "use it or lose it" appears to be a flip way of addressing such concerns, there is solid thinking behind it. As described in Chapter 4, when vaginal muscles contract more (due to orgasm or regular Kegel exercises, or both), they retain muscle tone. So most practitioners encourage women to have regular orgasms (through sexual intercourse or through masturbation) and to continue with Kegels.

Depletion of estrogen also impacts other parts of a woman's genitalia. The clitoris may become smaller and less sensitive to touch, and the vagina can narrow and shorten. Estrogen levels also have ramifications throughout the cardiovascular and nervous systems, creating changes that can affect a woman's sexual responses as well. For instance, restricted blood flow to the vulvovaginal area is associated with a change in the pH of the vagina and in vaginal secretions. Some women may experience a burning sensation after their partner's ejaculation because the pH level in their vaginas is not acidic enough to neutralize the alkalinity of the seminal fluid. Restricted blood flow may also account for uterine cramping that bothers some women during and up to 24 hours after orgasm.

Circulating estrogens trigger the release of neurotransmitters as well as neuroreceptors for serotonin and norepinephrine. When estrogen levels are too low, nerve impulses may be numbed; in fact, many menopausal women report numbness, clothing intolerance, and touch avoidance. Since touch is critical in human sexual response, a woman's willingness to have sex can be severely affected if she experiences such menopausally related neurological symptoms.

Many of these symptoms abate after hormone replacement, and your physician should discuss this with you if you're considering HRT.

If physiological reasons for diminished desire are ruled out, you and your physician may begin to consider the personal/sexual relationship in which you're involved. Each woman's level of sexual desire is different and is strongly affected by the changeable emotional climate between her and her partner.

The Totality of Sexuality

Human sexual response is an intricate, complex process. In terms of the physiology of sex, there are many neurological components to desire, and scientists believe that estrogen interacts with neurotransmitters in the brain. So it stands to reason that estrogen loss will cause changes in a woman's sexual response due to changes in her brain chemistry.

Often, we tend to view sex in narrow terms. As psychotherapist and sex therapist Wendy Schain points out, sexual behavior "is not just a penis in the vagina. It is a whole range of seductiveness, of fantasizing, of connecting in romantic nongenital ways, of connecting in romantic genital but not penetrative ways. So much of that can be altered by both hormonal changes and what happens to the androgens [male sex hormones] in menopause. It is likely that testosterone [an androgen] drives libido in both men and women, and part of our androgens do stem from our ovaries. So we need to measure not only FSH and LH, but we need to get an idea of which serum androgens are present exactly in women and which, when depleted, tend to give sexual dysfunction." The woman and her physician can then proceed to tailor a therapy to her particular hormonal milieu.

Desire: Hormonal or Psychological?

Physicians report that menopausal women and their partners often erroneously blame sexual problems on interpersonal difficulties. Fortunately, there is now more awareness in the medical community about addressing the sexual physiology of menopause. It makes sense to first rule out any physical cause for your sexual difficulties before looking into possible emotional issues. (See "Trouble-Shooting Problems with Sex" on page 105.)

Awareness about the physiology of desire will hopefully mean that women will stop blaming sexual problems on their psychological makeup, a tendency that places an additional burden on us when we're already feeling overstressed from the pressures of midlife, family, and menopause.

In a similar way, men experiencing erectile dysfunction used to believe there was something psychologically "wrong" with them. Before the 1970s, physicians thought most impotence was psychogenic in origin. Now, most causes of erectile dysfunction have been found to be organic, with very few cases that are purely psychological in origin.

Peggy Golden, formerly of UCLA's Human Sexuality Institute and a certified sex therapist in private practice with her husband, Joshua Golden, M.D., notes that multiple physiological effects are caused by lack of estrogen. Many of the body's autonomic systems are affected—basal metabolism rate, the cardiovascular system, and the neurological system. "And, with those neurological losses, it only stands to reason that there will be losses of sensation at orgasm." Even gynecologists and endocrinologists, she maintains, are not well versed in the neurotransmission of sexual response. It's a mistake to paint a rosy picture, telling women that they will not feel any different, when in fact, *everything* will feel different after menopause.

So if you consult your gynecologist or your general practitioner about problems with sex during menopause, it is important that you be heard. If your physician has sensitivity in this area, he or she will most probably follow these steps in your treatment:

• Carefully take a sexual history.

- Assess whether you are in menopause and what effect this is having on sexual function.
- Do a pelvic exam to try to detect any anatomical causes of sexual dysfunction.
- Recommend hormone replacement therapy, if indicated; discuss other options.
- Provide information on sex after menopause.
- Refer you for professional help if psychological conditions, such as depression, anxiety, or marital problems, appear to be contributing to your problem.

Psychological Losses

As much as we might try to deny it, we need to acknowledge that there are sexual changes associated with menopause. Given the effect on our sex organs, sex may become quite different. A woman may not feel like making love as much, or in quite the same way, for a variety of reasons.

If we understand the ways in which we've used our sexuality prior to menopause, we can gain some insight into our midlife sexual shift. "We use sex to communicate," says Dr. Schain, "and we also use it as a way of avoiding communication. We use it to achieve intimacy, but also as a way of *avoiding* intimacy. Not infrequently, I will encounter women [in my practice] who really use their husbands as they would a dildo—almost like a human masturbatory experience, with no interaction. These are the women who can't kiss their partner."

On the other hand, Dr. Schain explains, some people who have sexual dysfunction *don't* engage in sex because "for them it is an opening of a whole cascade of feelings that they need to keep tightly controlled. For some people, having sex is really an affirmation of being caught up in life and being full of feeling. That is too threatening for them, so they avoid sexual activity as a way of avoiding feelings.

"Other people avoid feeling by *being* sexual. That's all they feel in the moment, and so nothing else exists—it enables them to block out other feelings. When I do an evaluation of a sexually dysfunctional individual, I always try to get an idea of the ways in which they use sex. For some, it's an antianxiety device, for others, an antidepressant.

"What is real important is, if sex has been one of the ways in which a person has handled psychological issues and coped, and it is now no longer available to them [or no longer available in the same way], they may get incredibly depressed because of that."

Of course, some women, for many emotional reasons in addition to physical discomforts like vaginal dryness, turn away from sex almost completely.

These are the women, according to Dr. Schain, "who see menopause as another window of opportunity—that is, finally, to close it. Clearly there are women who have waited for a real good reason to say to themselves, 'I don't have to do this anymore. I don't *want* to do this anymore. It really doesn't feel good.' After years and years of not having fulfilling sexual relationships, having sex be either emotionally or physically painful, and now having it be unbearable, they are finally able to say, 'Absolutely not.' Their discomfort, along with some probable changes in erectile function and performance with their partners, allows them finally to fade out . . . and not feel guilty."

I talked with one man in his 60s who knew all about menopause. That's because when his wife went through it nine years ago, she stopped having sex with him—and hasn't slept with him since.

That sort of scenario would seem like a terrible loss to women like Jane, who cherish the pleasure and joy sex brings to her and her husband. Of course, points out Dr. Schain, "The people for whom it's a loss don't let it [the loss] happen." Women who are troubled by the sexual changes of menopause need to discuss their concerns with their practitioners, who can then help them come up with a viable course of action.

What Causes Sexual Dysfunction?

Types of sexual dysfunction usually fall into two groups: strictly physical complaints (dry vagina, loss of sensation) and loss of desire. The two are inextricably bound together, however, and tend to influence and affect each other.

Physical remedies exist for vaginal dryness, recurrent yeast infections, and bladder problems. For most of these conditions, estrogen is the treatment of choice. Likewise, hormone replacement can successfully remedy loss of libido. If HRT doesn't change a woman's diminished desire, however, other possible causes need to be investigated. First of all, consult the list "Trouble-Shooting Problems with Sex: The A's and D's." If, after careful examination and history-taking, your practitioner suspects the causes are related to relationship difficulties, he or she may refer you and your partner to a therapist.

♋   ♋   ♋

TROUBLE-SHOOTING PROBLEMS WITH SEX: THE A'S AND D'S

According to certified sex therapist Karen Lee Fontaine, most practitioners look for the following causes of lack of desire, one of the most common sexual dysfunctions.

The A's

Alcohol—Although many people still think of alcohol as an aphrodisiac that releases inhibitions, its action is mainly as a depressant.

Anger—If you're angry with your partner, being close and intimate and making love are furthest from your mind.

Anxiety—Although some people use sex as a way to relieve anxiety, most need to feel some degree of relaxation in order to feel interested in sex.

The D's

Drugs—Prescription and/or "recreational" drug use may be the culprit in loss of desire. Many drugs, such as antihypertensives and beta-adrenergic blockers, act against the neurological sexual response, while recreational drugs such as cocaine or marijuana may cause a variety of physical and psychological symptoms that interfere with or distort sexuality.

Depression—This clinical condition has the effect of dulling just about any good feelings a person may have. Behind many cases of depression are unresolved anger or trauma from the past or a chemical imbalance. Depression can be treated by psychotherapy alone or in conjunction with taking antidepressants.

Deliberate control—Partners often use sex, especially withholding of it, as a way to control or establish power over the other.

Dissociation—One or both partners may cut off their sexual feelings in order to avoid dealing with their emotions in general.

Check: diet, smoking, drug or alcohol use/abuse, medications

Check: self-image

Check: relationship difficulties

Check: partner's slowing down

Check: fatigue level, especially if you have young children (or even teenagers) still at home

Source: Karen Lee Fontaine, M.S., certified sex therapist.

↩   ↩   ↩

Getting Help for You and Your Partner

It's possible that just by relaxing a little about sex, you and your partner can find a new equilibrium. For instance, Gloria A. Bachmann, M.D., suggests "changes in the sexual script," which can entail sexual exchange with or without penile penetration, a warm bath before sex, or having sex in the morning when you are less fatigued.

As for physical aids, water-based nonhormonal vaginal lubricants can be helpful in temporarily alleviating vaginal dryness. These are usually short-acting, can be applied right before intercourse, and may even be incorporated into foreplay. Long-acting moisturizers that contain polycarbophil are also available. These lubricants adhere better and can provide more extended relief.

Estrogen-based vaginal creams or estrogen-impregnated intravaginal rings can actually restore layers of cells in the vagina and replenish urinary tract tissues. Both must be prescribed by a physician.

When it is clear that your sexual problems go deeper than the physical effects and could benefit from therapy, your physician may refer you and your partner to a marital counselor. Many marital therapists are also certified sex therapists, and you may decide that this could be helpful.

Usually, a sex therapist works with couples on a short-term basis, 10 to 12 sessions. Karen Lee Fontaine describes the process for treating lack of desire:

"Typically, inhibited sexual desire is the result of anger or conflict in the relationship. We do the two-pronged approach, giving both insight and behavioral assignments. What's nice about this is that sometimes when you do behaviors, attitudes change and when attitudes change, behaviors change. So if you get them both going, I think changes occur more quickly.

"After a getting-acquainted and history-taking session, which takes one to three hours, I start out having the couple [go home and] do a lot of nongenital touching, a lot of massage, learning how to touch each other's bodies and talk about it—what feels good and what doesn't. And that builds a lot of intimacy, besides getting some physical affectionate needs met. After that, depending on the couple's values, we may include mutual masturbation and then gradually add breast touching and genital interaction.

"In addition to this, I typically ask the couple to have three 'home play' times during the week. With busy schedules, I sometimes schedule clients every other week. They have a hard time finding free time, which is kind of sad. Some of them have put sex as number 76 on the list, *in pencil,* and it's the first thing to get erased.

"But I also assign what I call sofa sessions, which are 20 minutes long, of talking undisturbed, if possible. They can't run the family business during that time, nor can they fight. Often I will assign topics depending on their histories or what comes up in a session. So there will be topics about intimacy or subjects they're afraid to talk about, or where they want to be a year from now. I have them keep journals and logs so we can put it all together."

Fontaine doesn't push couples to delve deeper if they're reticent: "I try and work as short term as possible and deal with what the clients want to deal with. I'm not going to try and create problems or say, 'Aha! Here's a problem that's not bothering you, but let's make sure it does so we can cure it.'"

The same rule might apply to our attitudes toward sex and menopause: Let's not create a dread of problems that may not occur. But, if we have a plan for getting help, it will make dealing with sexual difficulties that much easier. This philosophy can also help guide you as you move into Chapter 6.

Best Resources

Therapists

American Association for Sex Educators, Counselors and Therapists (AASECT)
P.O. Box 5488
Richmond, VA 23220-0488
www.aasect.org

This interdisciplinary professional organization, comprised of sex educators, counselors, and therapists, as well as physicians, nurses, social workers, psychologists, and others, is directed toward promoting understanding of human sexual and healthy sexual behavior. One of AASECT's services, available by written request along with a #10 business envelope, stamped and self-addressed, is to provide lists of referrals of sex therapists or counselors in your state.

Note: It is *never* appropriate for a therapist to suggest exercises that involve a sexual or touching encounter between client and therapist. If this is suggested by your therapist, terminate the session and call your state's Board of Quality Assurance office to register a complaint.

Books

Sexual Turning Points: The Seven Stages of Adult Sexuality, by Philip Sarrel, M.D., and Lorna J. Sarrel. Lippincott Williams & Wilkins, Philadelphia, 1966; 366 pages; $52.95.

Human Sexual Response, by William Masters and Virginia Johnson. Little, Brown and Company, Boston, 1966; 366 pages; $46.00.

These two books by noted pairs of researchers impart much knowledge about sexuality from a scientific as well as a humanistic point of view. Good background reading. (Sarrel's book is currently out of print. You may want to check with your local bookstore for ordering, or simply check out a copy from the library.)

Books on sex abound in today's bookstores. Such titles as *Hot Monogamy, How to Drive Your Man (or Woman) Wild in Bed,* and *How to Make Love to One Another* attest to our cultural quest for the exciting and ultimately fulfilling sex life. I have found two books that relay a more sensible tone: *Sex Over 40,* by Saul Rosenthal, M.D. Jeremy P. Tarcher/Putnam, Los Angeles, 1989; paperback, 288 pages; $9.95; and *Romantic Massages,* by Anne Kent Rush. Avon Books, New York, 1991; paperback, 145 pages; $11.00. The latter has tasteful line drawings interspersed throughout accompanying the chapters, for example, "Breakfast in Bed."

CHAPTER SIX

Menopause and Beyond: Should You Be Worried?

I couldn't see why I needed to take medication for a disease that I didn't have. My nurse practitioner sort of scared me. She told me my vaginal tissues were thinning, and that if I didn't take HRT now, the usual scare stuff would happen: heart disease and osteoporosis. I also have a migratory joint condition that's probably stress-related. I've tested negative on every rheumatoid panel, every systemic lupus panel. They never figured out what it was and put me on some kind of anti-inflammatories, but the rheumatologist I went to said, "You absolutely have to take estrogen to prevent osteoporosis." I feel as though I'm being horribly pressured by everybody. What about my mother and everyone else who didn't take it? I'm very physically active. My mother at 78 was straight as a stick and never lost an inch of height. I don't believe I have a predisposition to any of those things.
Penelope, 52

Healthy women don't like to take pills.
Janis Luft, N.P., M.S., Mt. Zion Faculty Practice, University of California, San Francisco

We all make decisions to try to avoid risks. And there's no question about it, that's the smart thing to do. However, the decision not to use [hormone replacement] therapy is known to increase certain risks also. And that's an important thing to remember: The decision *not* to take treatment is as important a decision as the decision to use therapy.
Paul G. Stumpf, M.D., reproductive endocrinologist, Jersey Shore Medical Center

111

As you learned in earlier chapters, a woman may complete her menopausal transition with mild, moderate, or severe symptoms. If she's had intense hot flashes or other disruptive signs, she most likely will have sought treatment. Once through the transition, though, many women report feeling a renewed vigor and redirection of their energies. Having successfully weathered the discomfort, they may now feel uncomfortable with what their doctors are recommending, as Penelope was. Their menopause may not have been particularly difficult, they may feel perfectly healthy, and yet they're being told that they should consider hormone replacement therapy.

Thanks to mounting knowledge about the aging process and postmenopausal health, you have an opportunity to think ahead, to sort through your options, and to ensure better health and vitality in your later years. Whatever your experience with the climacteric, you've got another 25, 30, or 40 years to plan for!

Concern Versus Worry

One of the reasons menopause can be so confusing is that so many differing recommendations are offered by practitioners. One recent survey of 200 Los Angeles area gynecologists revealed that 86 different hormonal regimens were being offered to their patients!

Are women being pressured into hormone replacement therapy? Is Western medicine using scare tactics to exhort women to save their bones and their hearts by taking replacement hormones for an indeterminate number of years?

The answers depend on whom you're talking to. Let's start with a review of the scientific realities: When the ovaries cease the release of eggs, the level of circulating estrogens in the body declines sharply. This has consequences for many of the body's vital systems. Estrogen is an essential element in the bone remodeling process, in elevating the body's levels of HDL (good cholesterol), and in keeping genital and urinary organs toned.

Many public health experts, epidemiologists, and doctors look at the rapidly increasing numbers of aging women in our population, and they are concerned about the trends. "The majority of us will probably live through our 70s into our 80s. And one out of two of us is going to end up in a nursing home," says Janis Luft, N.P., M.S., of the University of California, San Francisco's Mt. Zion clinic. "Most of us end up in nursing homes because of cardiac problems or because of osteoporosis and fractures. The overwhelming majority of those women who have fractures, who break their hips in their 70s, are not able to return to an independent lifestyle."

So, in response to the question "Should you be worried?" I would answer, "Not necessarily worried, but concerned." You need to keep abreast of your body's changes and pay attention to the signals of trouble along the way. As with all the other symptoms surrounding menopause, it's important to realize the consequences of changes in your heart, bones, and bladder and to have some sort of plan to deal with them. "The take-home message that I want all women to know," asserts Luft, "is that there are a number of health concerns after menopause that—irrespective of your decision of whether or not to choose hormone replacement therapy—need to be addressed in some fashion."

In this chapter, you'll become familiar with the major challenges and long-term health risks of postmenopause:

- cardiovascular disease

- osteoporosis

- vaginal atrophy and bladder problems

- memory loss and brain function

You'll learn the risk factors for each and what you can do to lower your chances of becoming a statistic associated with the two "silent" diseases of old age: heart disease and osteoporosis. (These are called "silent" because the diseases' early developmental stages often occur without overt symptoms.) You'll also learn about hormonal and behavioral solutions to the discomforts of vaginal atrophy and urinary incontinence, lifestyle changes you can incorporate into your routine, and screening tests you should have on a regular basis to help in your own health care monitoring.

Heart Disease: Be on the Alert

Cardiovascular disease is also a woman's disease—it is not a man's disease in disguise.

> Carolyn Murdaugh, Ph.D., R.N., professor, acting scientific
> director, National Institute of Nursing Research, and chief of
> the Laboratory for the Study of Human Responses to Health
> and Illness, National Institutes of Health

By now, you may be hearing the message: Heart disease, not cancer, is the number one killer of American women. Combined deaths from heart attack and other blood vessel diseases have reached an annual rate of 500,000 women. Breast cancer, another major killer, takes approximately 46,000 women's lives, while lung cancer claims 41,600. Despite all the public health messages during the last several years, most American women are still fairly relaxed about heart disease. The commonly shared conception is that men are the ones who need to worry about heart disease. This is partly because few women develop cardiovascular disease before midlife.

But menopause changes all that, just as it changes so many other physical realities. When women do start having heart attacks (about a decade later in life than men do), they're more likely to die from the first attack than are men. That's because the progress of heart disease is less monitored in women, tends to be undertreated, and therefore is more progressed when a woman first reports symptoms to her doctor, or suffers her first attack. For instance, a well-known 1987 study found that men underwent coronary artery bypass surgery *four times as often* as did women, independent of age, presence of disease, or abnormal test results. In other studies, physicians surveyed believed that angina (chest pain) is a benign symptom in women because many women with chest pains do not have coronary artery disease.

Risk Factors and Menopausal Changes

One reason women don't worry as much about heart disease as men do is that we have not been educated about the dangers, probably because up until menopause, we enjoy more protection from heart disease because of our estrogen levels. Also, as the above studies reveal, the medical establishment seems to have had a blind spot when it comes to heart disease in women.

Concurrent with losing estrogen protection, another consequence of aging kicks in about the same time as menopause: The metabolism slows down and body fat gets redistributed. Using DEXA (dual energy X-ray absorptiometry) to measure body fat distribution, a group of researchers publishing in the *American Journal of Clinical Nutrition* compared distribution of body fat in pre- and postmenopausal women. What they found is that fat distribution in postmenopausal women tends to resemble the pattern found in men—they get thicker around the waist. Before menopause, body fat in women often distributes more around the hips than the middle, giving a more pearlike shape. The thicker middle, or so-called apple shape, often has been used as a predictor for cardiovascular disease risk. What are some of the other risk factors?

In Chapter 2, you took the "Heart Test for Women" and got a pretty good idea of your risk profile from the factors mentioned. What that test did not emphasize was the ways in which you could deal with the changeable and unchangeable risk factors embedded in it. The following information provides you not only with a risk factor assessment, but ways to deal with your particular health liabilities.

Unchangeable Risk Factors

Age
The older you are, the more likely you are to get heart disease.

Gender
After menopause, your risk of heart disease starts to equal that of men because of loss of estrogen.

Race
African Americans have a greater risk of heart disease than Caucasians because their blood pressure levels tend to be higher.

Family history
If a close relative has had heart disease, your likelihood of getting it increases.

What to do
Learn your family health history. Keep track of this and other vital factors and discuss them with your doctor. If your family history warrants it, make sure you're being closely monitored by your doctor. Ask whether exercise is advisable, what type, and how much of it you should do.

Although you cannot change your age, gender, or race, there may be changeable risk factors more under your control.

Changeable Risk Factors

Smoking
Because it constricts blood vessels, makes the heart beat faster, and increases blood pressure, smoking increases a woman's chance of heart attack two to six times compared to women who don't smoke.

High blood pressure
More than half of women over 55 have high blood pressure (140/90 or more on several separate readings), which increases risk of stroke and heart and kidney disease.

High blood cholesterol
High levels of blood cholesterol cause fatty deposits, called plaque, which narrow the arteries. Blood flow slows down and can eventually become blocked. See the box on page 117 listing normal cholesterol levels.

What to do
Stop smoking; monitor your blood pressure and take measures to lower it (exercise, diet, medication if your doctor prescribes it); lower your total cholesterol levels (change to a high-fiber, low-fat

Normal Cholesterol Levels

Total Cholesterol: Less than 200 milligrams/deciliter (mg/dl).

High-Density Lipoprotein (HDL): More than 35 mg/dl.

Low-Density Lipoprotein (LDL): Less than 130 mg/dl.

- Between ages 45 and 55, the average woman's total blood cholesterol rises to 223–246 mg/dl.

- The ratio of total cholesterol to HDL is considered equally important as the total cholesterol number. See Table 6-1 on page 124 for information on cholesterol ratios.

diet; ask your doctor about medication if you have hereditary high cholesterol). Take steps to raise HDL or "good" cholesterol levels: Exercise regularly, and consider hormone replacement therapy. Studies in men have shown that for every 1 percent decrease in cholesterol, there's a 2 percent decrease in risk of heart attack. Unfortunately, we do not have exact figures of decrease in risk for women because studies have not yet been conducted in this area.

Additional Risk Factors

Diabetes is a greater predictor of coronary heart disease (CHD) in women than in men. Diabetic women should be very carefully monitored for early signs of heart disease.

Lifestyle, career, personal relationships, and roles women play may also affect their risk of heart disease, although these are not solely independent indicators. For instance, some studies have documented a correlation of good health with marriage and employment. Poor health has been associated with role dissatisfaction, decreased social support, and/or a nonsupportive boss at work. This means that if you are the sole support of your family or primary caregiver for children and aging parents, you may be at risk for more health problems, including stressors that relate to heart disease.

Prevention Options

Perhaps we should demand some colossal well-controlled trials before we let the genie of universal preventive prescription escape from the bottle.

> Jan P. Vandenbroucke, writing in "Viewpoint," The Lancet 337 (April 6, 1991)

Larger studies are not necessarily better studies. . . . When the benefits of oestrogen [British spelling] therapy for the individual are so well established, hypo-oestrogenic women with premature ovarian failure, osteoporosis, hot flushes, dyspareunia, urinary frequency, or a family history of cardiovascular disease will not want to wait for the results of the colossal trials advocated by a well androgenised male.

> Jean Ginsburg et al., writing in response to Professor Vandenbroucke's letter, The Lancet 337 (May 11, 1991)

Should you replace your estrogen?

Estrogens have been in use for more than 40 years now, but the debate over their proper use shows no signs of being resolved. While the indication of estrogen for prevention of osteoporosis is sanctioned by the federal Food and Drug Administration, its use for prevention of cardiovascular disease is not. In practice, however, many clinicians already prescribe HRT as a preventive for heart disease. This clinical practice is based on results of studies, including the highly regarded Nurses' Health and Leisure World studies, that have demonstrated that women on estrogen experience a 50 percent reduction in ischemic heart disease (heart disease and stroke caused by narrowing of the arteries). It is possible, however, that since progestins blunt the rise of HDLs with estrogen, the beneficial effects of replacement therapy are considerably compromised by the addition of progestins to the therapy regimen.

Unopposed estrogen (estrogen given alone, without a progestational agent) is not usually given to women who have intact uteruses because it can cause too much growth of the uterine lin-

---

HRT Combinations in PEPI Trial

1. Unopposed estrogen (estrogen given alone).

2. Estrogen plus a cyclic progestin (a synthetic form of progesterone is added the last 12 days of taking the estrogen, thus mimicking the body's estrus cycle).

3. Estrogen plus a continuous progestin (a smaller dose of progestin is given each day, to minimize the side effect of monthly bleeding).

4. Estrogen and a micronized progesterone (a natural progesterone in a very fine powder, thought to be more easily absorbed by the body), taken 12 days a month.

5. A placebo (one group takes pills containing no hormones, to act as controls for the other groups).

---

ing, leading to a proclivity toward uterine cancer. Until researchers can ascertain the effect that progesterone has on lipids and other blood factors, HRT will not be approved by the FDA as a prescription for cardiovascular disease prevention.

The Postmenopausal Estrogen-Progestin Interventions Trial (PEPI) has recently yielded results which help to define the role of combined hormone therapy. Begun in 1991, the trial enrolled 875 participants, who were randomly assigned to receive one of the combinations listed in the box above. The first report issued in November 1994 revealed that each of the four hormone regimens lowered a woman's risk of heart disease significantly. In the mid-1990s, researchers hoped that upcoming studies would further refine the cardiovascular benefits of estrogen, as well as the best combinations in which to take it. However, as the disappointing results of the Heart and Estrogen/Progestin Replacement Study (HERS), released in August 1998, revealed, scientists and doctors may have been relying on the wrong assumptions about estrogen and heart protection.

Until more specific information from PEPI and other studies becomes available, women who are on HRT should have their cholesterol levels checked at least annually, if not every six months. Women without uteruses can take estrogen and not worry that it will build up endometrial tissue, as is the risk in nonhysterectomized women. (Without progesterone to trigger shedding of the uterine lining thickened by estrogen, a woman can be at greater risk for uterine cancer.)

Most clinicians do not recommend that a woman who has an intact uterus take unopposed estrogen, but some women may opt for this course of action. Several women I talked with did not like the bleeding, bloating, and mood swings associated with monthly progestins. They agreed with their physicians to have yearly endometrial biopsies so that they could take estrogen only. Women considering this option, however, are advised to heed the results from a second PEPI report, released in February 1996, which further underscored the risk of taking estrogen alone. The women receiving only estrogen without a progestin were much more likely to require an unscheduled biopsy (66.4 percent compared with 7.5 to 11.7 percent in the various combination groups, and only 8.4 percent in the placebo group). Another option might be to ask your physician about natural progesterone, available in a cream or oil base from compounding pharmacies such as Women's International Pharmacy (listed under "Best Resources" in Chapter 4), which reportedly does not have the same side effects as synthetic progesterone. Not much clinical study of natural progesterone has been done, so be prepared to learn that your physician may not have evidence of its efficacy in protecting the uterus. Monitoring the endometrium, through a biopsy or endovaginal ultrasound, makes good sense whether you are on HRT or not, so talk with your doctor about incorporating this screening into your annual checkups.

In the meantime, the American Heart Association (AHA) has changed its stance regarding traditional HRT to fight heart disease. New recommendations released in May 1999 by the AHA in collaboration with the American College of Cardiology call for physicians to consider using statins, drugs that are specifically designed to lower cholesterol, instead of hormones for heart disease in postmenopausal women. If women have other problems such as bone loss that generally dictate hormone replacement, then a combination of statins and hormones might be called for. If you are taking hormones to lower your risk of heart disease, you may want to talk with your doctor about this issue.

Nonhormonal prevention options

At a gathering of pre- and postmenopausal women last year in the California coastal town of San Luis Obispo, one woman transformed the renowned real estate maxim, "Location, location, location" into a panacea for midlife health: "Exercise, exercise, exercise!"

Regular exercise is important for a variety of reasons: It lowers the levels of LDL (low-density lipoprotein or "bad cholesterol") in your blood, imparts a general sense of well-being, and helps you maintain muscle strength and flexibility. A six-month study of 101 postmenopausal women reported in the February 1994 issue of *Obstetrics and Gynecology* found that those who exercised moderately three times a week improved cardiorespiratory fitness and lowered their LDL levels, thus affording them more protection from cardiovascular disease than their sedentary counterparts. Women in the study who exercised *and* took estrogen appeared to have the most protection, because the hormone actually increased levels of HDL (high-density lipoprotein, the "good" cholesterol).

Postmenopausal women I interviewed who seemed the happiest were those who were active. Their activities took many different forms: Many women walked daily; others jogged, attended aerobics classes at their local senior citizens' center, or were members of square dancing clubs. Los Angeles naturopath and acupuncturist Janet Zand points out, "You can have the most perfect diet in the world—eating only fresh, whole foods and getting plenty of good herbs and nutrients—but if you're not exercising, that nutrition is not being fully utilized."

To be beneficial to your heart, exercise should be consistent— three to four times a week, for at least 20 to 30 minutes at a time. And it should be aerobic. *Anaerobic* exercise such as weight lifting would not apply here (although weight-*bearing* activities are important in preventing bone loss). If you haven't been an exerciser, talk with your doctor about how to begin. If you've never exercised much, or are returning to it, remember that it's important to start slowly and build up your endurance gradually. And follow the principles of "warm up, cool down" to ease your muscles before and after a workout.

Exercise alone won't guarantee a healthy heart. Combining regular exercise with a sensible eating plan may be the best insurance. The healthiest diet for your heart is one with very little fat, although the recommendations vary on what percentage of your diet fat should comprise. The American Heart Association advises limiting daily intake of fats to a maximum of 25 percent of total calories. Nutrition programs such as the Pritikin Longevity Center's go even lower—10 percent calories from fat. Mounting evidence on the link between dietary fat and certain types of cancer (colon, breast) is also prompting the National Cancer Institute to recommend a maximum daily total fat intake of 20 percent of calories.

If you opt to make changes in your diet, keep in mind that lifestyle changes like this can be difficult. As with an exercise program, your chances of maintaining a healthy regimen are improved if you make changes gradually. Beware of any crash dieting plans. Choosing a sensible weight loss program such as Weight Watchers, which emphasizes healthy eating and gradual weight loss, can improve your chances of success. Or you may decide to devise your own diet plan. Assess what you normally eat by keeping a log over a period of one week to 10 days. Then educate yourself about the differences between saturated and unsaturated fat versus cholesterol. Consider where you could painlessly eliminate some of the fat from your diet. Don't be unduly strict with yourself, because that is a sure way to set up a feeling of deprivation. For instance, if you love Italian food, avoid cream-based sauces, veal, and meatballs, but experiment with different varieties of pastas and sauces made with vegetables sautéed in a small bit of olive oil. Treat yourself to a "light eating" recipe book—but make sure to determine whether the use of oil in the recipes is really low.

Finally, as another prevention option, look for ways to reduce the stress in your life. Regular exercise can go a long way toward this goal, but also consider creating peaceful times during your day, even if they're relatively short in duration. Women who are the primary caregivers for children or aging parents must be especially careful to set aside time for themselves each day. Without that vital hour or so to replenish our resources, we serve ourselves and others less well.

Whatever your plan for keeping your heart and blood vessels healthy, use the checkup recommendations in Table 6-1 to observe proper monitoring and screening for early detection of disease.

Your Bones: Constantly Changing

Because our bones are hard on the outside, we tend to see them as static, unchanging. But bone is not an inert material; it's constantly forming, breaking down, and re-forming. As old bone is broken down and new bone builds up, metabolites from that process leave markers in the blood and in the urine. Testing for these markers has become increasingly widespread, due to the proliferation of new biomarker tests on the market. However, women should not accept these tests as substitutes for bone density testing for diagnosis of bone loss, cautions Dr. Robert Lindsay, an endocrinologist and president of the National Osteoporosis Foundation. These tests "are definitely not ready for prime time," he said. "There's too much interindividual variability and intraindividual variability. If you send morning urine away [to the lab], you'll get a different result than if you send evening urine away. So I'd be very cautious about using any of these tests." Biomarkers can be useful, he continued, when used to monitor calcium levels after osteoporosis treatment has begun, to assess if the drug is working.

Bone loss is a process that varies with the individual. In the general population, bone loss begins in about the mid-30s. In the first five to seven years after the menopausal transition, the rate of bone loss speeds up, to anywhere from 1 to 3 percent per year.

Of course, we all start out with different skeletons. A woman who has been fairly athletic might have big, strong bones and lose bone at a slower rate. She also possesses better reserves and perhaps can tolerate more of a loss. A woman who starts out with smaller bones at menopause and loses at a more rapid rate needs more protection.

Why do you need to be concerned about bone loss? It can lead to osteoporosis, in which the bone becomes so porous that it's brittle and breaks easily. Osteoporosis is the "fragile bone" disease,

Table 6-1   Checkup Recommendations for Heart Health

Blood Pressure:	Yearly, if in the normal range (120/80 is normal; 140/90 is high). Twice yearly or even monthly if you are on a modification program (such as weight loss or antihypertensives).
Blood Lipid Levels:	• Yearly, if in the normal range. • Twice or four times yearly, if in borderline category. • Monthly, if on a modification program (such as weight loss or medication to lower cholesterol).
Total Cholesterol:	Less than 200 mg/dl—good. Between 200–239 mg/dl—borderline. 240 mg/dl and above—high risk.
HDL (high-density lipoprotein):	50 mg/dl or above—very good. 35–50 mg/dl—good. Under 35 mg/dl—increased risk.
LDL (low-density lipoprotein):	Less than 130 mg/dl—good. 130–159 mg/dl—borderline. 160 mg/dl and up—high risk.
Triglycerides:	20–140 mg/dl—normal range. 140–190 mg/dl—above normal. 190 mg/dl and up—high risk.

Ratios of HDL to total cholesterol and of HDL to LDL are as important as the total cholesterol numbers. According to the American Heart Association, the desirable ratio of total cholesterol to HDL is 4:1. A "good" range would be 200 mg/dl total cholesterol to 50 mg/dl HDL. The Arizona Heart Institute and Foundation has refined these ratios for women, and offers these ranges for low, moderate, and high risk for heart disease:

Divide Total Cholesterol by HDL number to get your ratio of risk:

$$\frac{\text{Total Cholesterol}}{\text{HDL (high-density lipoprotein)}} = \text{Ratio of Risk}$$

Example: 200 mg/dl total cholesterol, 50 mg/dl HDL: 200 ÷ 50 = 4

Lowest Risk: Ratio of 2.9–3.6 total cholesterol to HDL (*Example:* total cholesterol of 200; HDL of 93 = 2.15, very low risk).

Moderate Risk: Ratio of 3.7–4.6.

Highest Risk: Ratio of 4.7 or higher.

Stress Treadmill: Performed in a hospital or clinic setting, this test is used to diagnose blocked arteries. The problem is that a treadmill test is rarely useful unless disease is already present. Blood pressure and blood lipid monitoring are much more useful as preventives.

Source: AHA, Arizona Heart Institute and Foundation, Phoenix, Arizona.

and for women who experience fractures, it's painful, debilitating, and ultimately life-threatening. For women now entering menopause, the news is much better than it was two generations ago. We know more about retarding bone loss, and many recent studies of new compounds have shown promise of not only halting bone loss but actually rebuilding bone.

Bisphosphonates have become an important tool in treating osteoporosis. These compounds have been shown to both inhibit bone breakdown and increase bone density in well-conducted studies. One of the bisphosphonates, Fosamax, manufactured by Merck, has been widely prescribed since its FDA approval and market release in early 1996. However, many women have reported severe digestive discomfort when taking Fosamax. The manufacturer recommends that patients take their pills first thing in the morning with a full glass of water and that they stand for at least a half hour after taking it. A more convenient weekly tablet (70 mg) is now available. Other types of bisphosphonates are now being tested; one is risedronate by Procter & Gamble.

Another class of drugs, the selective estrogen receptor modulators, or SERMs, has also shown activity against osteoporosis. Evista, or raloxifene, was recently approved for the prevention of osteoporosis. The excitement about this drug stems from revelations that in addition to bone protection, it also produces changes in blood lipids that may be favorable. Researchers are moving quickly to find alternatives to HRT for heart and bone health. You can stay current on developments with new drug treatments by asking your doctor or accessing one of the Internet sites listed at the end of Chapter 1.

Risk Factors and Disease Prediction

The following chart provides a simple questionnaire to assess your personal risk factors for getting osteoporosis. You should take your results with a grain of salt, however. Researchers caution that the risk factors are only about 50 percent predictive of who will actually get osteoporosis and suffer serious fracture. The main use of such a risk factor chart is to get a general sense of your bone health, after which you can proceed deliberately and at your own pace to come up with bone loss prevention strategies.

∾ ∾ ∾

Assessing Osteoporosis Risk

Y   N

———   ———   1. Female?

———   ———   2. Early menopause? (Natural menopause before 45 or surgical menopause.)

———   ———   3. Caucasian or Asian?

———   ———   4. Chronically low calcium intake? (1,000 mg daily recommended premenopause; 1,500 mg daily after menopause.)

———   ———   5. Chronic lack of physical activity?

———   ———   6. Underweight?

———   ———   7. Family history of osteoporosis?

———   ———   8. Cigarette smoker?

———   ———   9. Excessive use of alcohol?

The more times you answer "yes," the higher your risk of getting osteoporosis. Take this questionnaire with you to your doctor. If you answer "yes" to family history of osteoporosis or being a smoker, these are considered more critical than just being female.

Source: "Osteoporosis, Cause, Treatment, Prevention," NIH Publication No. 86-2226; revised May 1986; National Institute of Arthritis and Musculoskeletal and Skin Diseases.

∾ ∾ ∾

In addition to the risk factors cited in the above questionnaire, the National Osteoporosis Foundation suggests that you may be at risk for developing osteoporosis if you or an immediate family member have broken a bone as an adult or if you are taking high doses of thyroid medication or steroids for conditions such as asthma or arthritis.

Who Should Have a Bone Scan?

If you are concerned, because of your race, frame, build, former health habits, or family history, that you may be at risk for osteoporosis, you may want to discuss scheduling a bone scan with your gynecologist or primary care physician. The majority of bone scans are performed using DEXA (dual energy X-ray absorptiometry). This is a noninvasive 20-minute procedure, performed while you lie on the X-ray table with your knees elevated. The X ray is usually taken of four lumbar vertebrae (see Figure 6-1) and of the neck of the left hip, a common site of fracture in the elderly with porous bones (see Figure 6-3). The accompanying printouts (Figures 6-2 and 6-4) illustrate how the computerized X-ray machine graphs bone density and compares it to the norms of the female population in the appropriate age range. Some experts recommend a different type of bone scan called quantitative computerized tomography, or QCT. The advantage of QCT is its ability to measure 100 percent of the spongy bone marrow in the spine, and detect very small changes. For this reason, QCT is the method used by NASA to measure bone loss of astronauts in the space program. The spongy bone is more susceptible to changes from a stimulus, such as estrogen loss or drug therapy, than the thick outer bone. However, you get a slightly higher dose of radiation with QCT. And since DEXA is now the worldwide standard, your bone density

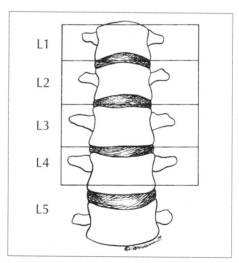

FIGURE 6-1 Example of bone scan of lumbar spine. *Illustration by Carol Beckerman*

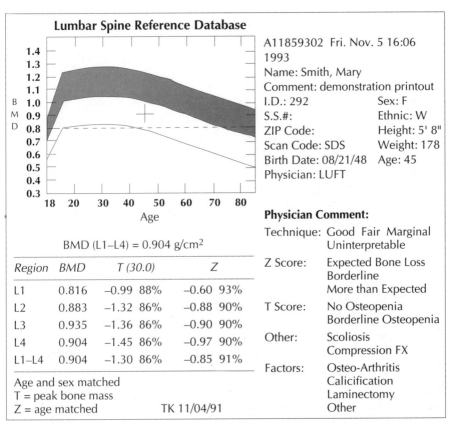

Lumbar Spine Reference Database

A11859302 Fri. Nov. 5 16:06 1993
Name: Smith, Mary
Comment: demonstration printout

I.D.: 292	Sex: F
S.S.#:	Ethnic: W
ZIP Code:	Height: 5' 8"
Scan Code: SDS	Weight: 178
Birth Date: 08/21/48	Age: 45
Physician: LUFT	

BMD (L1–L4) = 0.904 g/cm^2

Region	BMD	T (30.0)		Z	
L1	0.816	–0.99	88%	–0.60	93%
L2	0.883	–1.32	86%	–0.88	90%
L3	0.935	–1.36	86%	–0.90	90%
L4	0.904	–1.45	86%	–0.97	90%
L1–L4	0.904	–1.30	86%	–0.85	91%

Age and sex matched
T = peak bone mass
Z = age matched   TK 11/04/91

Physician Comment:

Technique:	Good Fair Marginal Uninterpretable
Z Score:	Expected Bone Loss Borderline More than Expected
T Score:	No Osteopenia Borderline Osteopenia
Other:	Scoliosis Compression FX
Factors:	Osteo-Arthritis Calicification Laminectomy Other

FIGURE 6-2 Computer printout of a bone density scan. The "T" column gives the percentage of bone mass for the individual woman. The "Z" column compares her bone mass to other women her age.

measurements will be compared to the World Health Organization averages for women your age. Talk with your ob/gyn and your radiologist to see what they think is best for you.

Consensus regarding candidates for regular bone scans has yet to be reached. Unless a woman already exhibits signs of osteoporosis, most insurance companies and medical plans do not reimburse for this procedure. If you are interested in finding out a baseline of your own bone health, you may have to pay for the scan out of pocket (prices range from $200 to $300). According to Janis Luft, the following are some women who might consider a bone scan:

- Menopausal or postmeno-
pausal women who are at
risk for osteoporosis (see
"Assessing Osteoporosis Risk"
checklist on page 126).

- Premenopausal women who
have not menstruated for
years due to excessive exercising, anorexia nervosa or
other eating disorders, or
unexplained causes. (These
women have been estrogen
deprived before the average
age of menopause and thus
may have suffered substan-
tial bone loss prior to the age of 50.)

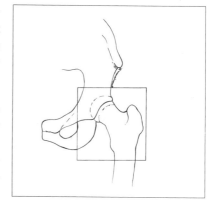

FIGURE 6-3 Area of left hip scanned by DEXA. *Illustration by Carol Beckerman.*

- Women who have chronically taken steroids for the treatment
of asthma or other conditions. (Steroids hasten bone loss.)

- Women who have gone through radiation therapy for cancer
of the bone and other cancers.

- Women who have been bedridden for long periods of time (remember that astronauts lose bone when they are not subjected
to the pull of gravity).

- Menopausal women who want to have a baseline of their bone
density in order to help make a decision about whether to take
hormone replacement, or women who have decided against
HRT and want to monitor the condition of their bones after
menopause.

While most guidelines for bone density scanning do not recommend the test until age 65 or older, many women do not want
to wait that long for a baseline. Even women who do not have the
specific risk factors identified in the earlier questionnaire may request a scan. Dr. Paul Stumpf has been "humbled" by the amount
of hidden bone deficiency uncovered in his own patients. Women
for whom a scan did not seem necessary have actually turned out

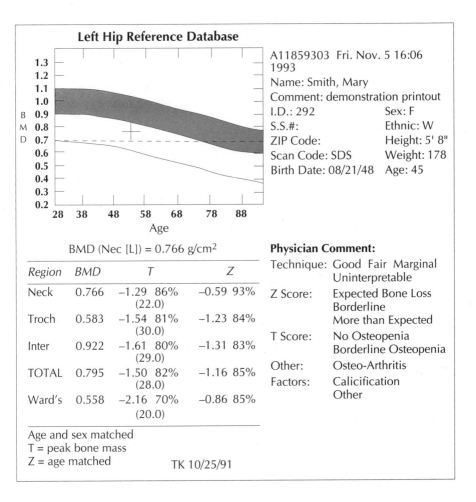

FIGURE 6-4 Computer printout of bone density graph.

to have bone loss warranting some kind of prevention therapy—and that's a big difference.

The bone density scan will allow you and your doctor to determine the percentage of bone loss, if any, and gauge whether the bone loss warrants treatment. Some bone scan computer programs also express bone loss in terms of "deviation from the norm." World Health Organization guidelines for establishing a diagnosis of osteoporosis are two standard deviations from the norm for all women your age. If you are one standard deviation below the norm, your chances of developing osteoporosis are slightly increased. Having another scan in a year of two might be a good idea. If you are right at the norm, you could wait longer to have another scan. If you've lost a higher percentage of your bone density and are two standard deviations below normal ranges, your physician will most probably recommend hormone replacement to stop the bone loss. Research and development are proceeding swiftly in this area—as seen with the approval of new osteoporosis drugs like Fosamax and Evista. A study recently published in the *Annals of Internal Medicine* revealed that low-dose (0.3 mg) conjugated equine estrogen, the form used in Premarin, in combination with calcium and vitamin D supplementation was effective in preventing bone loss. The lower dose of estrogen also resulted in fewer side effects, such as breast tenderness and stomach discomfort, associated with the standard 0.625 mg doses. Every year women will have more options available to them.

Other Prevention and Treatment Options

For women unable (because of contraindications) or unwilling (because of fears of cancer and side effects) to take estrogen, other options exist.

Gail A. Greendale, M.D., assistant professor of medicine at the University of California, Los Angeles, works with menopausal breast cancer survivors who are, for the most part, precluded from taking hormone replacement. Pharmaceutical alternatives to hormones for preventing osteoporosis for these women include calcitonin, also called salmon-calcitonin, given by injection; calcitriol, an injectable form of vitamin D; and a slow-release fluoride. (Fluoride has been found to improve bone density, but earlier forms also increased the number of fractures.)

In addition, Dr. Greendale and many other public health advocates urge women to prevent falling—an obvious but sometimes overlooked commonsense approach to preventing fractures. To prevent falls, follow these suggestions:

- Get regular exercise. It's been shown that if you're reasonably fit, you're less apt to lose your balance and fall.

- Be aware of any medications you may be taking that affect your sense of balance. This is one of the major causes of falling in older adults.

- Conduct a home-safety assessment to decrease the danger of slipping on rugs, electrical appliance cords in walkways, or overwaxed floors.

Finally, as with heart disease prevention, assessing your diet is really important. The same basic principles apply: A low-fat, high-carbohydrate diet is best, with lots of fruits and vegetables. Adequate sources of calcium are also important (see Appendix A, "Calcium-Rich Foods"). If you find that you're not getting at least 1,000 mg of calcium a day from your diet, a calcium supplement is strongly recommended. As women age, they absorb calcium less well. After age 60, a woman cannot readily absorb calcium carbonate, for example. Researchers recommend taking another form of calcium such as calcium citrate, which is more readily absorbed, and ingesting supplements between meals so that levels of calcium remain more constant. Vitamin D, from daily exposure to sunshine or from dietary or supplemental sources, is also necessary for proper calcium absorption.

Finally, be careful not to overdose on calcium. If you take more than 1,500 mg a day (the maximum recommended for a woman not on HRT), excess calcium may cause kidney stones because the kidneys will have to work overtime to excrete the calcium that's not absorbed.

Urogenital Health

"A lot of women really haven't been told the story," maintains Janis Luft, "about atrophic vaginitis and bladder changes after menopause." Because the vagina and urinary system are estrogen-dependent, changes are to be expected during and after menopause. Chronic vaginal pain is a common consequence of post-menopausal vaginal dryness and tissue atrophy. Your physician will first need to determine the exact cause of your vaginal pain and can prescribe various concentrations of vaginal estrogen creams. It takes about three months for tissues to grow another layer of cells, but often such therapy can be short term.

Maintaining continence can also become a problem after menopause, because the bladder and urethra are less toned without estrogen. The treatment of choice for these conditions is usually estrogen, but Luft is now participating in a study that teaches women behavioral techniques for controlling incontinence. These include the practice of consciously resisting the urge to urinate to decrease the number of times a day it happens. The theory is that the urge to urinate can become self-fulfilling and that by constantly fixating on urination, a woman unconsciously "trains" her bladder to respond. These resistance exercises, combined with Kegel exercises (see Chapter 4), which are good for both the vagina and bladder floor, represent some progress in treating incontinence nonhormonally.

Estrogen and the "Brain Drain"

Each year, more evidence accrues about the association between estrogen and brain function. As they enter the perimenopause, many women complain of problems with "fuzzy thinking" and memory loss. "That's probably the one thing [about estrogen loss] that I have to grieve the most," comments Bonita D. Zisla, M.F.C.C., M.A., a therapist in Los Osos, California. "I've always been somebody with a nearly photographic memory. I've relied on my memory for many things. The information's still there, but I can't find it as quickly. That's the big one for me. I had worked through a lot of body issues, but I hadn't worked through the brain issues: 'Okay, what am I going to do when I'm dumber?'"

Zisla's colleague Susan Swadener, Ph.D., R.D., a nutritionist who teams with Zisla to lead eating and body image workshops for women, reminds us that there are "estrogen receptors in the brain, as well as in the bone and the breast."

HRT is showing promise as a possible treatment to delay the onset of symptoms of dementia and Alzheimer's. A large study sponsored by the Women's Health Initiative is now under way. Called the Women's Health Initiative Memory Study, or WHIMS, the multicenter study will eventually include 8,300 women who will be followed for six years and be assessed annually for cognitive function. The study will be comparing HRT to placebo to see whether HRT reduces the incidence of dementia in women aged 65 and older.

The approach to health risks after menopause involves two parts: getting information and devising a plan. If you've yet to go through menopause, you should consult some of the tips in Chapter 2, "Entering Menopause: Where Do You Stand?" because good health involves many of the same principles throughout life.

The next two chapters address the emotional challenges of menopause and beyond, and give you ways to deal with the emotional risk factors you may encounter.

Best Resources

Resources for staying abreast of new information on women and heart disease, menopause, and midlife health include the following.

Studies to Watch For

National Center for Complementary and Alternative Medicine
As part of its expanded program to test alternative and complementary therapies, NCCAM continues to fund studies at various university sites. Many of these relate to concerns of menopausal women, such as "The effects of soy consumption on estrogen in women," "Hormonal responses to a low-fat, high-fiber, and soy diet," and "Lifestyle and ovarian function in midlife women." More information about breaking studies can be obtained by accessing NCCAM's home page through www.nih.gov.

PEPI
The Postmenopause Estrogen-Progestin Interventions Trial was finished in mid-1994. The first report reaffirming cardiovascular benefit was published in November 1994. The second report confirming the safety of adding a progestin to the estrogen regimen

was published in February 1996. A third report on osteoporosis was released in late 1996, and others have followed.

WAVE, WELL-HART, and ERA trials

The National Heart, Lung, and Blood Institute (see "Best Resources" in Chapter 1 for Web site address) is supporting several ongoing trials, including the Women's Angiographic Vitamin and Estrogen (WAVE) trial, the Women's Estrogen/Progestin and Lipid Lowering Hormone Atherosclerosis Regression trial (WELL-HART), and the Estrogen Replacement and Atherosclerosis (ERA) trial. All are looking at whether estrogen, alone or in combination with progestins and vitamins, can lower lipids that lead to artery blockage (atherosclerosis) and heart attack or stroke.

Women's Health Initiative

This is a huge, broad-ranging study of multiple factors (diet, exercise, and more) in 55,000 to 60,000 postmenopausal women aged 50 to 79.

One section of the WHI is a 10-year prospective study of 25,000 women, with the goal of determining whether HRT prevents heart disease and whether it increases risk of breast cancer. Another is the Women's Health Initiative Memory Study (WHIMS), which will look at the effects of HRT on development of dementia in women 65 and older.

How to participate in a study

If you would like to participate in a study on postmenopause, contact the nearest university teaching hospital, or log on to the National Heart, Lung, and Blood Institute's Web site (see "Best Resources" in Chapter 1) and click on the Women's Health Initiative.

Associations

National Osteoporosis Foundation
1232 22nd Street N.W.
Washington, DC 20037-1292
(202) 223-2226
www.nof.org

The NOF has many publications on prevention and treatment of osteo-porosis, some of which are available on their Web site. Also included on the Web site are an on-line catalog of educational materials, and information you can print out on "Medications and Osteoporosis."

National Institute on Aging (NIA)
NIA Information Center
P.O. Box 8057
Gaithersburg, MD 20898-8057
(800) 222-2225
www.nih.gov/nia

Printed materials can be ordered from the NIA either by phone or on-line; sample titles include "Osteoporosis: The Bone Thinner" and "Sexuality in Later Life."

American College of Obstetricians and Gynecologists
P.O. Box 96920
Washington, DC 20090-6920
www.acog.org

Brochures and pamphlets published by ACOG are available on a number of menopause-related subjects, including hormone replacement and heart, bone, and urogenital health. These can be obtained through your gynecologist or by writing or telephoning the ACOG office or E-mailing the ordering person listed on their Web site. You can access a Physician Directory, Patient Education section, and Maintaining Wellness section on their Web site. You can also search their brochure titles and get up to five copies of each mailed to you free of charge.

Your local chapter of the American Heart Association is an excellent resource for all kinds of free materials on keeping your heart healthy. Along with information pamphlets, they also offer low-cholesterol booklets and tips on proper monitoring of heart conditions.

Your local chapter of the American Lung Association is a good source of materials on smoking cessation. Their approach is commonsense and very supportive.

Books

"Osteoporosis: What You Can Do to Prevent It, Plus New Techniques for Managing the Disease," Chapter 17 in *Menopause and Midlife Health,* by Morris Notelovitz, M.D., Ph.D., and Diana Tonnessen. St. Martin's Press, New York, 1994; 480 pages; $17.95.

Stand Tall! The Informed Woman's Guide to Preventing Osteoporosis, by Morris Notelovitz, M.D., Ph.D., with Marsha Ware. Bantam Books, New York, 1985; paperback, 208 pages; $7.95.

CHAPTER SEVEN

The Body/Mind Connection: Menopause and Emotional Stress

I thought I was starting to go through something the last few years—my periods were getting irregular and I had more menstrual discomforts. Then I got a hot flash and thought, Aha! This must be it. When I got the FSH test results confirming menopause, I thought, "Wow! I'm in menopause!" I felt like calling all my women friends and celebrating!

Charlene, 49

This wasn't a happy year for me. My mother died and then I went into menopause. Maybe because both these events happened together, I became really depressed. I felt old, that I was going to die next and what was the use of trying to do anything? Since being in the support group, though, I've been able to separate some of the grief about my mother from my feelings about my future. And now, you know, I can't wait to turn 51!

Susan, almost 51

Does going through menopause mean you'll experience an emotional crisis? Many premenopausal women fear this is so; however, research has found that the opposite is true. Menopause itself is not a precipitator of major crises or depression, so you need not brace yourself for the worst. And yet, you *will* notice real physical changes, which can influence the feelings you have about menopause and growing older. Body and mind are interconnected, as

Eastern disciplines have believed for thousands of years, and as Western medicine now recognizes. Stresses in the body can affect the mind and emotions. Having a context in which to view these shifts can help you decide on a course of action.

Physicians no longer view menopause as solely a physical change. Testament to this view can be found in physicians' journals (for example, *Postgraduate Medicine* and *American Medical News*), in articles urging physicians to acknowledge and treat the menopausal patient as a whole person. As with any complex set of physical changes, menopause elicits emotional responses. Withdrawal of estrogens made in the ovaries has consequences for almost every system in the body, even the brain.

In addition to the emotional ramifications of estrogen loss, a woman must deal with the emotions surrounding another loss: the end of her reproductive years. This closure can be further complicated by our society's views of aging, and by a woman's own attitudes and experience. For instance, the end of childbearing may be a relief to someone who's raised four children and wants to get on with her life, but it signifies a time of mourning for the woman who wanted a child but never had one. Thus, the personal and societal context in which menopause occurs can be as significant or even more significant than physical symptoms.

The "givens" of menopause are that it *will* happen, and that physiological changes occur. But menopause is not merely a set of biological changes; it is an interweaving of the biological with the psychological. Its physical manifestations can bring about psychological symptoms directly—as with mood swings, anxiety attacks, and mental confusion—and can also trigger emotional responses, such as sadness, regret, and depression over getting older.

Just as with other pivotal events in a woman's life—marriage, childbearing (and rearing), divorce—menopause can prompt a host of reactions, ranging from the joy that Charlene talked about, to the grief Susan experienced. For women like Susan, the convergence of two important life events, her mother's death and her own "change of life," put her into a temporary tailspin.

In this chapter, we'll explore the physical and psychological stressors of menopause. You'll get an idea of how to assess your own stress level, as well as how to acquire some tools to strengthen your coping strategies when you're feeling overwhelmed.

How Women Feel About Menopause

Why do some women embrace menopause joyfully while others undergo depression and sadness? For some, the climacteric transition is just plain uncomfortable physically. For others, hormonal changes seem to trigger anxiety and mood swings. Menopause does not happen in a vacuum; it occurs within the context of a complex life. Having lived some 40 to 50 years, each woman brings a wealth of experiences to this juncture in her life. In addition, says nurse practitioner Pamela Pilate, "We bring certain coping skills to this point in our lives, and for whatever reason, some of those coping skills are not going to work."

A woman's expectations about her menopause may also influence her experience of it to some degree. Studies of perimenopausal and menopausal women are revealing some interesting conclusions. One Canadian study, conducted by researchers at St. Michael's Hospital of Toronto, found significantly greater psychological distress among perimenopausal women as compared to menopausal women. The researchers found that 113 women in the period right before menopause scored higher on indexes for anxiety, hostility, depression, and paranoid attitudes than did the 146 women who were menopausal. A well-known study by Professor of Psychiatry Karen Matthews of the University of Pittsburgh, which looked at the symptoms women experienced through menopause, revealed that natural menopause "did not have negative mental health consequences for the majority of middle-aged healthy women." These two studies could be seen in an additional light when placed side by side. Could it be that for perimenopausal women, the hormone fluctuations leading up to menopause made them more susceptible to emotional swings than women who had already "reached the other side"?

Despite observations by Matthews and others, some women do experience emotional upheaval during menopause. Their distress can be brought on by a range of hormonal, physical, and emotional causes, which we'll discuss next.

Emotions and Stress During Menopause

As scientists begin to investigate menopause more closely, they've dispelled some of the long-held myths about menopause, beliefs that often influenced women's expectations about their own impending menopause. But here again, as in other areas of medical research, there is disagreement about what menopause actually causes and what it doesn't.

Among more progressive physicians, the consensus seems to be that menopause does not cause depression. A woman entering menopause may be suffering from an underlying depression that can surface or be exacerbated because of other complaints. There are several theories about the factors contributing to adverse psychological symptoms at menopause.

Biologic changes

Changes in the body's hormone "mix" because of declining estrogens have been reported to affect neurotransmitters in the brain. Endorphins, natural opioids (opiatelike chemicals) made in the body, are also associated with estrogen. Replacing estrogen after menopause often increases that opioid activity, producing an antidepressive effect.

"Domino theory"

Menopause may cause extreme cases of hot flashes, night sweats, and interruption of REM (rapid eye movement) sleep, the level of sleep necessary for deep rest and dreaming. Lack of REM sleep can easily set up a temporary unbalance—ask any sleep-deprived new parent! Sleep deprivation, in turn, causes irritability, fatigue, and difficulty thinking and concentrating.

Psychosocial factors

Society's views toward aging women can promote negative experiences of menopause. Women's fears about loss of control over their bodies can also cause negative responses. "The real crisis for women is not hot flashes but coming to terms with the fact that they are no longer 28," points out Alice Rossi, a sociologist at the University of Massachusetts who studies the changes of middle age.

Is Depression a Given?

There are physical reasons for many of the so-called psychological symptoms of menopause, and most researchers agree that the onset of clinical depression in middle age is more likely attributable to psychosocial causes. Here it is important to remember that there is a difference between clinical depression, which often requires treatment to be resolved, and transitory grief over the changes signaled by menopause. The box on page 144 lists some of the signs of clinical depression, which can be treated by various methods including antidepressants, psychotherapy, or combinations of both.

If you or family members have noticed several of these signs in you, it is important to consult with a certified and knowledgeable therapist.

What You're Facing with Menopause

What are some of the issues that might normally trigger sadness or grief at menopause?

Having to face one's mortality

The finality of menopause often causes women to confront their own mortality. "When we were young and summers were endless, there was plenty of time," reflects Judi Powers, M.F.C.C., director of the Center for Women's Health with Brotman Hospital in Culver City, California. "But now we are being brought up short."

Confronting the realities of aging

Our culture, unlike those of China or Africa, does not revere age—it idolizes youth. "We've always gotten the message in this culture that it's not okay to be old," says Carol Barme, co-therapist with Judi Powers of the Women in Midlife groups at Brotman Hospital. "So the first signs you have that you're getting old, you want to keep that to yourself." This attitude may be changing, however, as large numbers of the boomer generation move collectively into their fifth decades.

Facing the end of one's reproductive years and/or childlessness
Marty, 43, had just begun to consult a fertility specialist for help in conceiving when she got the startling news that she was, in fact, menopausal. After a few months of confusion and bereavement,

Some Signs of Clinical Depression

- Changes in sleeping or eating patterns *not attributable to menopause or other obvious causes.*

- Sudden increase in or intolerable levels of anxiety, anger, or despair.

- Feelings of extreme isolation, loneliness, or unhappiness.

- Self-destructive urges (suicidal thoughts and feelings) or addictive behavior (such as abuse of alcohol or drugs).

- Change in sex drive. (This is a tricky call during menopause, and may require a consultation with your doctor.)

- Inability to function properly or to cope with ordinary routines.

- Marked changes in mood from up to down, or prolonged periods of mood swings from euphoric to depressive.

Source: Health Research Group, Department of Health and Human Services.

she and her husband started adoption proceedings. Many women are childless by choice, but others may have to deal with the reality that any children they have will not be biologically theirs.

Dealing with real physical discomforts

It's no fun to be sick, and if your body is putting you through hell, it's hard to feel cheerful. After 50, women are more likely to be dealing with a number of chronic physical complaints—urinary incontinence, diabetes mellitus, joint or arthritis pain. To the degree that these conditions are controllable, a woman can expect to have some relief. But feeling under par can do a lot toward prompting depression. The remedy in such cases is to make sure you've explored all the options for care. Finding a way to ameliorate physical discomfort is sure to improve your mood.

With all these factors operating simultaneously, it's no surprise that women have a lot of emotions surrounding menopause. Finding expression for her feelings about menopause with her doctor, spouse, or friends will be more helpful for a woman than trying to repress or "stuff" them down. To the degree that a woman is able to divulge her fears and sadness in a safe environment (one in which her confidences will not be used against her), she may feel freer to go to the next stage after menopause—a renewed interest in her own life priorities.

How Menopausal Changes Cause Stress

Despite the new openness concerning menopause, it can still be a shock when an individual woman realizes she has reached this time in her life. Judith LaRosa, Ph.D., deputy director of the National Institutes of Health's Office of Research on Women's Health, recalls that even as a scientist she at first didn't grasp what was going on. "My mother told me she went through menopause at 55. So I thought, well, that gives me some time. I think what she meant was that she finished going through it at 55. Anyway, I couldn't figure out what was going on with my lipids [levels of fat in the blood]. I happen to have very good lipids, and my husband is a lipidologist at George Washington University. But suddenly my

HDLs [good cholesterol levels] were going down from 93 to 83. And here I was, going to all these medical meetings talking about the effects of estrogen on lipid levels, and it finally dawned on me: It was starting!" LaRosa went to her gynecologist, who took an FSH and LH blood test and confirmed she was in menopause. She already had a plan, and had decided to go on HRT. But for that initial time, she wasn't prepared for the change.

Change can be good or bad, or a combination of both. But whether a change is positive or negative, it brings stress. A woman in menopause faces physical changes and new emotional realities. Although Eastern and Western disciplines disagree in their interpretations of stress response and their prescriptions for how to deal with it, recognition has grown in both disciplines that body and mind are intertwined, working together—or against each other.

When you enter menopause, stress is likely to be a factor, simply because of the new layer of change that's being added to your life. It can be helpful to understand what we know about response to stress before you think about ways to deal with it. The Western interpretation is based on research into the "fight-or-flight response," first identified by Dr. Walter Cannon in the 1930s. In response to threat, the body's sympathetic nervous system goes into action. The adrenal gland pumps out more epinephrine, which speeds up the heart rate and constricts blood vessels. The breathing rate increases, and the blood coagulation system is activated so that blood will clot more quickly in case of injury. For our earliest ancestors, these responses gave the body the jump start it needed to flee from a menacing animal or enemy—or to stand and fight—thus the label "fight or flight."

In our modern world, our bodies also respond to threat. The reactions, however, are much more complex than they were for our early ancestors. For instance, perhaps a coworker insults you in the hallway at work. You seethe, your heart beats faster, you're ready to fight. To physically fight your colleague is socially unacceptable, and even to argue with him or her (especially if the coworker is your superior) would be foolhardy in terms of keeping your job. So you say nothing. You finally simmer down, but on the way home from work you get stuck in a heavy traffic jam. You suddenly find yourself cursing the other drivers.

This accrual of stressful situations, without the accompanying release of physical energy, can lead to many problems, among them inappropriate or delayed responses to threat. Accumulated stress can also literally make a person sick. In Eastern philosophies, practitioners believe that such stress causes the body to build up certain toxins that must be released or they will block energy flow throughout the body.

While most of us associate negative stress with harmful body changes, it's also possible to "stress out" with too much good news. Marilyn, 62, remembers her menopause vividly: She was becoming a grandmother for the first time, a very happy event, but when she took on the duties of hostessing a baby shower for her daughter, her hot flashes increased and she got heart palpitations. Her doctor advised her to slow down and to get some regular exercise. Most things were going right in Marilyn's life. Why was she having a bodily response? It turns out that the main cause of stress is *change*—be it good or bad. Thomas Holmes and Richard Rahe, two social scientists who did research in the mid-1960s, identified a whole list of stressors in a person's life that, when they accumulate, can lead to more susceptibility to illness. The "Holmes/Rahe Social Readjustment Rating Scale" appears in the following list. Taking the survey gives you a window into the number of stressors in your life. Many women enter the climacteric in the midst of dealing with a number of stressful events. Although it's enlightening to add up the stressors, don't allow a high score to worry you. There is a lot you can do to lower your stress level.

☙   ☙   ☙

HOLMES/RAHE SOCIAL READJUSTMENT RATING SCALE

Life Event	Value*
1. Death of a spouse	*100*
2. Divorce	*73*
3. Marital separation or end of relationship	*65*
4. Jail term	*63*

(continued)

(*continued*)

Life Event	Value*
5. Death of a close family member	63
6. Personal injury, illness, abortion, or miscarriage	53
7. Marriage	50
8. Fired from work	47
9. Marital or relationship reconciliation	45
10. Retirement	45
11. Change in family member's health	44
12. Pregnancy	40
13. Sexual problems	39
14. Addition of new family member	39
15. Business readjustment	39
16. Change in financial status	38
17. Death of a close friend	37
18. Change to different line of work	36
19. Change in number of marital arguments	35
20. Mortgage or loan over $100,000	31
21. Foreclosure of mortgage or loan	30
22. Change in work responsibilities	29
23. Son or daughter leaving home	29
24. Trouble with in-laws	29
25. Outstanding personal achievement	28
26. Spouse begins or stops work	26
27. Starting or finishing school	26
28. Change in living conditions	25
29. Revision of personal habits	24
30. Trouble with boss	23
31. Change in work hours or conditions	20
32. Change in residence	20
33. Change in schools	20
34. Change in recreation	19

(*continued*)

Life Event	Value*
35. Change in church activities	*19*
36. Change in social activities	*18*
37. Mortgage or loan under $100,000	*17*
38. Change in sleeping habits	*16*
39. Change in number of family gatherings	*15*
40. Change in eating habits	*15*
41. Vacation	*13*
42. Christmas season	*12*
43. Minor violation of the law	*11*
TOTAL	————

* If your total score in the last 12–18 months is less than 150, you have only a slight chance of developing stress-related illness. If your score is between 150 and 200, you have a 50 percent chance of becoming ill because of stress. If you score over 300 points, you have an 80 percent chance of becoming ill due to stress. Remember that illness ranges from frequent colds to severe heart and kidney disease. Also remember that the scale is relative to the way you handle situations. Your mind is the determining factor in your level of stress and the way that it affects your body.

Source: Thomas H. Holmes and Richard H. Rahe, "The Social Readjustment Rating Scale." *Journal of Psychosomatic Research* 11 (1967): 213–218.

∾   ∾   ∾

Steps You Can Take

They've been called the "sandwich generation"—women squeezed between aging parents and children who haven't left home, and who are expected to be the caretakers of both. "For the women who are in this situation," notes Sonia Hamburger, director for faculty education at the University of California, San Diego's Menopause Clinic, "menopause could not be coming at a worse time." These are the women for whom the additional stressor of menopause, and all that it may signify in their lives, is the final straw. Therapist Bonita D. Zisla points out that "in the past, women tended to slow down in their lives at this point. They had fewer responsibilities, they were probably through parenting, a lot of things were completed for them. Not for us—we're busier, probably, than we were." In addition, she says, "we don't really have a context [for going through menopause]. I don't think any other women have really done 'the change' the way we have. So, as usual, we're the first wave."

As many health care and women's health group advocates point out, this crisis may actually furnish women with an opportunity. By "getting their attention," menopause may spur them into taking a closer look at their stressful lives and finding ways to become more emotionally healthy. One of the best ways to do that is to make time for relaxation, a little peace and quiet. This doesn't require leaving town for the week. It can be done on a daily basis, and incorporated into your routines.

Your first step is to identify your present and potential stressors. Next, determine if the source of your stress can be changed. Suppose, for instance, that your elderly mother wants to come to live with your family. You may not be able to afford full-time nursing care for her, and you may not feel comfortable refusing her request. So you add a new stress to an already stressful life. If such were the case, you would need to focus next on reducing your *response* to the stress. The following section provides a few suggestions.

How to Become More Relaxed

Herbert Benson, known for his work on the relaxation response, identified necessary elements for the relaxation response: a quiet place, a passive attitude, a comfortable body position, and a meditative device or focus for the person's attention. You can achieve this response in a number of ways. One is to practice deep breathing (see the box on page 151). Other methods include:

Yoga

The beauty of yoga, at least in its less athletic forms, is that you incorporate stretching, muscle toning, and deep breathing in one workout. Meditation often ends a yoga class, and the ability to relax into your breathing comes with practice. Check with your local yoga society, local YMCA, or community college for classes.

Aerobic exercise

Aerobic exercise, which should be done with a certified instructor, can help reduce your stress level as well. To get the maximum benefit, exercise at least 30 minutes at a time, three times a week.

Visualization

Visualization, or imaging, involves taking yourself through a kind of mental journey. In order to do this, find a quiet place and either sit erect or lie down comfortably. You may start by doing some deep breathing. Then imagine yourself in a pleasurable situation. You can think about your favorite spot outdoors, or achieving an award. Repeat to yourself, "I feel calm and content. It is a lovely day and I am at peace with myself."

How to Practice Deep Breathing

You may remember from Chapter 4 that deep breathing has been found to ameliorate hot flashes, so you could be doing yourself some double good with this one. Here's how:

1. Sit or lie down comfortably.

2. Inhale deeply and slowly through your nose.

3. Place your hand on your stomach to feel it expand as you inhale.

4. Then purse your lips and slowly and steadily exhale, until your lungs have completely deflated.

Repeat this exercise 10 times, two to four times a day.

Meditation

Meditation can be done either alone or in a class. Transcendental Meditation (TM) is one of the best known methods.

Biofeedback

Biofeedback is a technique for controlling the autonomic (involuntary) nervous system by using monitoring devices that give you feedback—usually a sound or tone—when changes in blood pressure, brain waves, and muscle contractions occur.

Finally, find ways to treat yourself with respect and compassion. Accord yourself respect by seeking support and by setting aside time for yourself.

You are the best judge of what makes you feel better. It could be as simple as a long soak in the tub, a walk on the beach, or reading a good novel. Whatever course you take for being good to yourself, it's important to have things you do just for you. Now, more than ever, knowing how to relax will pay off when it comes to your health and well-being.

The Value of Support Groups

It's no secret that our emotions have a lot to do with how we handle events in our lives. There is even some scientific evidence that emotional well-being can influence the functioning of the immune system. That was the conclusion of some Stanford University investigators who found that breast cancer patients participating in support groups survived an average of 12 months longer than those who were not in support groups. What bearing does this kind of study have on menopause?

In group after group, as I listened to women talk about their experiences with menopause, one theme seemed to echo throughout: Isolation is the real enemy. When a woman feels as if she is alone and that no one understands what she is going through, she is likely to feel more frightened, more powerless.

Ann Kearney-Cooke, professor of psychology at the University of Cincinnati and therapist in private practice, believes that it's important for women in midlife to seek out support, just as new mothers do. "We have all sorts of rites of passage when you get engaged, when you get married, when you're going to have a baby," she points out. "It's very important to have a group that becomes that rite of passage, or some people who you share it [the experience] with. That is a very important experience, because when one woman names her reality, it really empowers another, and it also starts to contradict the distortions that you're seeing in the media."

Turning to other women can help lighten your load. Sharing jokes about chin hairs and doing Kegels can dispel depression about aging. Having fun with friends, finding alone time to keep a journal, or taking up painting or kayaking can release you from the burden of worrying about what comes next.

Our personal reactions to aging will most certainly be an important element in our adjustment to the changes of menopause. Once we are able to separate our views of ourselves from the societal constrictions, it may be that we can make more room to feel the pluses of this natural change in our life—the liberation that aging can bring. In the next chapter, we'll gain some insight into how women have approached the journey of their older years, using new energies to take them in some surprising directions.

Best Resources

Associations

National Self-Help Clearinghouse
Graduate School and University Center of the
City University of New York
365 5th Avenue, Suite 3300
New York, NY 10016
(212) 817-1822
www.selfhelpweb.org

This not-for-profit organization was founded in 1976 "to facilitate access to self-help groups and increase awareness of the importance of mutual support." The Clearinghouse position on self-help mutual support groups is that group members:

- feel less isolated knowing others share similar problems
- exchange ideas and effective ways to handle problems

- actively work on their attitudes and behavior to make positive changes in their lives
- gain a new sense of control over their lives and feel less overwhelmed by their problems

You can click on "Help Desk" on the Clearinghouse Web site and print out an order form for several publications, including:

How to Organize a Self-Help Group, $6.00

Self-Help Reporter, $10.00 for a one-year subscription (four issues a year)

Add $1.00 for postage on all orders.

Books

"Aging and Well-Being," in *Ourselves, Growing Older,* by Paula Brown Doress, Diana Laskin Siegal, and The Midlife and Older Women Book Project. Simon and Schuster, New York, 1987; paperback, 511 pages; $18.00.

The Relaxation Response, by Herbert Benson and Miriam C. Klipper. Avon, New York, 1976; paperback, 126 pages; $5.99.

Beyond the Relaxation Response, by Herbert Benson and William Proctor. Berkeley Publishing, New York, 1985; paperback, 192 pages; $4.99.

How to Meditate: A Guide to Self-Discovery, by Lawrence LeShan. Bantam Books, New York, 1986; paperback, 176 pages; $4.99.

Simple Abundance: A Daybook of Comfort and Joy, by Sarah Ban Breathnach. Warner Books, New York, 1995; hardcover, $21.00.

This book isn't for everyone, and some of the sentiments may be cloying, but there are enough useful nuggets—one essay for each day of the year—that you can take from it what you will and disregard the rest.

CHAPTER EIGHT

Integrating Change and Exploring Opportunity

I saw and see menopause as an incredible opportunity to be released from social and professional restrictions. . . . The truth of the matter is that my mind has changed. And I am now in the process of trying to get to know it, because it's not a mind that I expected. And I even worked to get those changes. My sense is to listen with curiosity for the changes.

Deena Metzger, 57, Los Angeles poet, teacher, therapist

Only when a woman ceases the fretful struggle to *be* beautiful can she turn her gaze outward, find the beautiful and feed upon it.

Germaine Greer, author of The Change, Women, Aging and the Menopause

No longer do the stereotypes of the hysterical midlife woman haunt us. To characterize their experiences of menopause and the years beyond, women often use terms such as *release, new directions,* and *renewed mental vigor.* As information about menopause becomes more available and accessible, women don't feel as anxious about the change of life. Although some wonder whether they'll feel more tired or uncomfortable as they go through the menopausal transition, or whether the side effects of HRT will be bearable, menopause is now acknowledged as a new beginning.

We've learned that a whole complex of hormonal changes occur during menopause that have both physical and psychological consequences—some immediate, some long-term. Knowing about the changes does not mean you won't experience any discomforts, but hopefully the preceding chapters have armed you with enough information to start assembling a health plan of your own.

Still, even with all the information in the world, women who have yet to go through menopause wonder what's in store for them. This is, after all, a very personal story as soon as it starts happening to you. Women I interviewed confessed feeling more uneasy about the *implications* of menopause than the actual physical transition. These feelings are naturally part of the journey, because menopause occurs at the gateway to the last third of life.

Although not true for every woman, and not of earth-shaking proportions for every woman, this time of physical change can be a catalyst for life review. Women can choose to reexamine their life choices or not; some may be pulled into reexamination unwillingly. What they find may be pleasing or not; and if not, may throw them into momentary upheaval.

It is this juncture of crisis and opportunity that this chapter addresses. Just as with the health plan chapters, this is not a prescription but rather an invitation to consider taking some time off for reflection, and to avail yourself of resources that can stimulate thinking about the meaning of this event for your life.

Menopause as Passage

Life is progression (hopefully) and change (certainly). How we adjust to and take meaning from these progressions and changes can determine our level of happiness, often measured by Western psychologists as "satisfaction," and denoted by Eastern practitioners as being "in balance."

Social scientists and psychological theorists have fashioned innumerable models for the various stages of adult life. For years, one of the most commonplace models for midlife women was that of going through the "empty nest syndrome." For the majority of women who had raised children, this was perceived as a time of mourning and role loss (Neugarten, 1968). But in fact, studies from the 1980s have shown that the majority of women actually look forward to the departure of their children (Reinke, Ellicott, Harris, Hancock, 1985). They see this time as one of personal growth and more personal freedom. A portion of the boomer generation have had children later in life, and are or will be going through menopause with adolescent and even younger children in the house. So if women aren't fearing moving on from parent-hood, what do they fear?

Perhaps apprehension about menopause is related to our gen-eral anxiety about change and our inability to know what the fu-ture holds. Along with such events as surviving a critical illness or having a loved one pass away, menopause is a time when a woman confronts her own mortality and is forced to take a more reflec-tive, realistic look at the meaning of her life. In the same way that the impending physical changes of menopause help her make healthier lifestyle choices, the aging process that menopause sig-nals helps her get her "psychic house" in order.

A woman may realize, "Hey, I'm getting older. I don't know if I want to continue [teaching school or traveling every week on business] until I retire. I'd like to find a way to do something I truly want to do."

Confronting change can be exciting as well as anxiety-producing. Women today, who entered the workforce 25 to 30 years ago in large numbers, are perhaps better equipped psychologically to deal with the fear and excitement of change. It's not illogical, though, for women to seek out the counsel of friends or a psychotherapist to guide them through these times of change.

"It's a good thing [menopause] only happens to older people with more experience," quips therapist Bonita D. Zisla, "because you have more things to draw on, with any luck at all. Wisdom tends to come as you get older. You know that you have survived and prospered through other times, so this is just another one of those—it just looks different than some of the other situations. I think of it as getting us ready for the great unknown, the great mystery."

Tackling the Tasks of Growing Older

Aging presents adults with a multitude of challenges. Certain reali-ties of getting older are not pleasant. No one really relishes consid-ering their own demise. I don't like the idea of my own mortality, nor do I particularly enjoy watching my body acquire more sags and lumps. Deena Metzger concurs: "There was a period where I watched the bone structure in my face change. And I watched it, and it was hard, and I didn't know how I would manage it."

But, it seems, aging has its rewards, its joys and satisfactions. "I'm not going to say that when I look down at my thighs and I see the thighs of an older woman and the belly of an older woman that it doesn't bother me so much," says Metzger. "But I think the major thing I've let go of is a certain kind of more adolescent ambition—I don't really care what the latest movie is, for instance. But the ambition is now going toward craft, my own accomplishment and sense of excellence."

Psychologists who study older people find that those over 50 are more comfortable with the interior world, with time, with the self. As people age, they attempt to resolve any conflicts between *interiority,* or turning inward, and *generativity,* or the sense that they have contributed something to future generations. Whether they've had children or not, women see menopause as a time for changes. They may have harbored dreams of what they would do "if they had the time." Well, it is entirely possible that menopause is capable of delivering that time. It might be just for a day, or part of every day, or a more sweeping change in routine, but women seem increasingly motivated to follow their own paths at this stage in their lives.

The media and literature are full of women who have made another start halfway through life—women who have finished raising their families and return to the university for a degree, who start a business on their own, or who continue in the same career but cut back on their hours to save more time for themselves.

Finding Your Path

Once we are past menopause we are all oddballs.
  Germaine Greer, The Change

It feels to me that there are really four stages [in a woman's life]: There's the girl, and then there's the mother, and then I think there's the woman in the world—the woman who educates herself and gives to the world, whether she gives as a volunteer for her charity or in terms of her grandchildren, or she actually becomes one of the leaders. It's still a sense of "Here is this wisdom and now I'm going to offer it." Then, I think there's another stage. And that's the stage when we pull in because something else is drawing us. And it is something about the spirit or silence. And I think people are really terrified of that. Because we have nothing in our society to prepare us for that pulling away.

Deena Metzger

Of course, not everyone wants to be an oddball or can be on the cutting edge of feminist thinking.

Still, there is something to the notion of listening to one's inner desires, of "marching to a different drummer." Some postmenopausal women speak of disengaging from a frenetic pace of life. Others are busier than ever, filling their time with volunteer and creative ventures. Whatever their direction, women in their older years are doing more of what suits them. Of course, their choices still need to be made in the context of such practical considerations as family obligations, monetary situations, and the like, but usually they find they have more freedom as they enter their fifth decade.

In eight-week group sessions conducted with midlife women, psychologist Ann Kearney-Cooke encourages women to become the "writers of their own stories." She leads them on guided "tours" of their girlhoods and young adulthoods to help them get in touch with their past and begin to carve out a future. Because we have no rituals for menopause (as we do for marriage and childbearing), Kearney-Cooke feels it's important that women make testament to one another. In this way, they can validate and encourage each other. "Instead of the red blood from your period," remarked one woman from her group, "there's the flowing of ideas that can occur."

"Once you can help women look at that, it [menopause] can be a very freeing time for them," reports Kearney-Cooke. Of course, you don't necessarily need a formal support group. You might simply get together informally with friends who are in menopause and talk about how your lives are progressing. Reading relevant books can also stimulate new ways of thinking about life stages and choices. (A recommended list appears at the end of this chapter.) Or you may find yourself with a renewed commitment to your religious faith, or turn to meditation for a deeper connection to your inner self. Many universities and local colleges offer courses in journal writing, an excellent tool for sorting out one's spiritual directions.

The habitual changes we all undergo, although scary and threatening at first, can engender a renewed *joie de vivre*. Germaine Greer names her last chapter in *The Change* "Serenity and Power" and talks about the depths of joy she has been able to experience since growing older. Gail Sheehy reports a time of what she has labeled "coalescence." Anthropologist Margaret Mead used to refer to the renewed energy of her postmenopausal years as "postmenopausal zest." No matter how exotic or simple our description of this unique season, it seems that life gives back even as it takes away. We might lose some of our agility (although thousands of physically fit midlife women of the 1990s seem to prove otherwise), but it's possible to gain a renewed purpose in life, a creative surge, a spiritual wisdom.

Menopause, during the transition, can be a bit of a bumpy ride. It may bring some of us to the brink of crisis. But out of crisis comes opportunity and the chance to evaluate important life choices in preparation for the next healthy and fulfilling quarter century of life.

My life is not tamed in any way. If anything, it is more courageous. I don't even think about things as being difficult or that I shouldn't do them. I want to do them and I do them. But, you know, I've come to a certain accomplishment and I know how I got there. So why be embarrassed by the things that got me there? —Deena Metzger

Best Resources

The Change, by Germaine Greer. Fawcett, New York, 1993; paperback, 432 pages; $14.00.

Menopause: The Silent Passage, revised edition, by Gail Sheehy. Random House, New York, 1998; paperback, 272 pages; $14.00.

Women of the 14th Moon: Writings on Menopause, Dena Taylor and Amber Sumrall, editors. Crossing Press, Watsonville, Calif., 1991; 325 pages; hardcover, $26.95; paperback, $14.95.

Calcium-Rich Foods

	Measure	Calories	Calcium (mg)
Dairy Foods			
Cheeses			
American, pasteurized	1 oz.	105	174
Blue	1 oz.	100	150
Cheddar, pieces	1 oz.	115	204
Feta	1 oz.	75	140
Mozzarella, made from whole milk	1 oz.	80	147
Mozzarella, w/part skim milk	1 oz.	80	207
Muenster	1 oz.	105	203
Parmesan	1 Tbsp.	25	69
Provolone	1 oz.	100	214
Swiss, pasteurized	1 oz.	100	219
Swiss	1 oz.	105	272
Cottage Cheese			
Low-fat (2% fat)	1 cup	205	155
Creamed (4% fat)			
Large curd	1 cup	235	135
Small curd	1 cup	215	126
Milk			
Skim	1 cup	85	302
1% fat	1 cup	100	300
2% fat	1 cup	120	297
Whole (3.3% fat)	1 cup	150	291
Buttermilk	1 cup	100	285
Dry, nonfat, instant	¼ cup	61	209

	Measure	*Calories*	*Calcium (mg)*
Dairy Foods			
Yogurt			
Plain, low-fat, w/added milk solids	8 oz.	145	415
Fruit-flavored, low-fat, w/added milk solids	8 oz.	230*	345*
Plain, whole milk	8 oz.	140	274

* Values may vary

	Measure	*Calories*	*Calcium (mg)*
Dairy Desserts			
Custard, baked	1 cup	305	297
Ice cream, vanilla, regular (11% fat)			
Hardened	1 cup	270	176
Soft serve	1 cup	375	236
Ice milk, vanilla			
Hardened, 4% fat	1 cup	185	176
Soft serve, 3% fat	1 cup	225	274
Seafood			
Oysters, raw, meat only, 13–19 medium	1 cup	160	226
Salmon, pink, canned, including the bones	3 oz.	120	167**
Sardines, Atlantic, canned in oil, drained, including the bones	3 oz.	175	371**
Shrimp, canned, drained, solids	3 oz.	100	98

** If bones are discarded, calcium is greatly reduced.

	Measure	*Calories*	*Calcium (mg)*
Vegetables			
Bok choy, raw, chopped	1 cup	9	74
Broccoli, raw	1 spear	40	72
Broccoli, cooked, drained, from raw, ½" pieces	1 cup	45	177
Broccoli, cooked, drained, from frozen, chopped	1 cup	50	94
Collards, cooked, drained, from frozen	1 cup	60	357

	Measure	Calories	Calcium (mg)

Vegetables

	Measure	Calories	Calcium (mg)
Dandelion greens, cooked, drained	1 cup	35	147
Kale, cooked, drained, from frozen	1 cup	40	179
Mustard greens, stems and midribs removed, cooked, drained	1 cup	20	104
Turnip greens, chopped, cooked, drained, from frozen	1 cup	50	249

Dried Beans, cooked, drained

	Measure	Calories	Calcium (mg)
Great northern	1 cup	210	90
Navy	1 cup	225	95
Pinto	1 cup	265	86
Chickpeas (garbanzos), cooked, drained	1 cup	270	80
Red kidney, canned	1 cup	230	74
Refried beans, canned	1 cup	295	141
Soy beans, canned, drained	1 cup	235	131

Miscellaneous

	Measure	Calories	Calcium (mg)
Molasses, cane, blackstrap	2 Tbsp.	85	274
Tofu, 2½" x 2¾" x 1" piece (about 4 ounces)	1 piece	85*	108*

*Values may vary, especially calcium content, depending on how the tofu is made. Tofu processed with calcium salts can have as much as 300 mg calcium per 4 ounces. The label, your grocer, or the manufacturer can provide more specific information.

Source: Home and Garden Bulletin 72, Human Nutrition Information Service, U.S. Department of Agriculture, 1985.

Comparison of Calcium Supplements

Note: The total milligrams of calcium in each tablet is not the amount your body will absorb. For each product listed below, the amount of *elemental* calcium it contains is also listed. This is the amount of calcium your body will actually absorb from the tablet, and the number you should use when figuring your daily intake of calcium. For women over 60, calcium citrate may be more easily absorbed by the digestive system.

Drug (Mfr. in parentheses)	Percent of Elemental Calcium	Amount of Elemental Calcium per Tablet	Dose (no. of tablets) for 1 g (1,000 mg) of Elemental Calcium
Calcium Carbonate 1,250 mg; Oyster Shell Calcium (Penta)	40%	500 mg	2
Os-Cal-500 (Marion)	40%	500 mg	2
Calcium Carbonate 1,250 mg w/200 IU vitamin D; Calel-D (USV)	40%	500 mg	2
Calcium Carbonate 625 mg w/125 IU vitamin D; Os-Cal 250 (Marion)	40%	250 mg	4
Calcium Carbonate, USP 650 mg (Lilly)	40%	260 mg	4

Drug (Mfr. in parentheses)	Percent of Elemental Calcium	Amount of Elemental Calcium per Tablet	Dose (no. of tablets) for 1 g (1,000 mg) of Elemental Calcium
Calcium Carbonate 500 mg; Tums (Norcliff-Thager)	40%	200 mg	5
Calcium Carbonate 420 mg; Titralac (3M)	40%	168 mg	6
Calcium Gluconate, USP 975 mg (Upjohn)	9%	88 mg	11
Calcium Lactate, USP 650 mg (Lilly)	13%	84.5 mg	12
Calcium Citrate; Citracal (Mission)	40%	200 mg	5

Sources: R. Don Gambrell, Jr., M.D., "Estrogen Replacement Therapy User Guide," Essential Medical Information Systems, Inc., Dallas, TX, 1989, pp. 60–61; and Kaiser Permanente Member Education Services, Sunset Center, Los Angeles, CA.

Dietary Recommendations for Health

Appendix C-1: American Heart Association Diet

The following diet tips are excerpted from "The American Heart Association Diet—An Eating Plan for Healthy Americans," and "How to Have Your Cake and Eat It Too," published by the American Heart Association (AHA) and available from your local AHA chapter.

The AHA eating plan is based on these guidelines, all aimed at reducing your blood cholesterol level. A high blood cholesterol level is associated with heart disease.

- Total fat intake should be less than 30 percent of all dietary calories. [Other plans call for a lower percentage.]
- Saturated fatty acid intake should be less than 10 percent of all dietary calories.
- Polyunsaturated fatty acid intake should be no more than 10 percent of all dietary calories.
- Monounsaturated fatty acids make up the rest of total fat intake, about 10 to 15 percent of total calories.
- Sodium intake should be no more than 3,000 mg (3 g) a day.

Fats Defined

Some fats are harmful to your heart, while others are not. Here are some general definitions.

Cholesterol

A fatty substance found in animal foods, such as meat, poultry, fish, egg yolks, milk, cream, cheese, butter, and other dairy products. Plant-derived foods contain no cholesterol.

Saturated fats

Contained primarily in animal foods including red meat and whole milk dairy products, as well as certain types of oils such as coconut and palm and palm kernel oils, used in commercially produced baked goods.

Monosaturated fats

Found in olive oil, canola oil, and in avocados; may actually reduce the blood cholesterol levels.

Polyunsaturated fats

Found in sunflower, corn, soybean, and safflower oils; may also reduce blood cholesterol levels.

Suggested Eating Selections

Meat, poultry, and fish

No more than 6 ounces per day of lean meat, poultry, or fish.

Choose from: fish (fresh, frozen, canned in water, or canned in oil and well rinsed), shellfish, chicken without skin, Cornish game hen without skin, turkey without skin, lean or extra-lean ground beef. One cup of cooked beans, peas, or lentils or 3 ounces of soybean curd (tofu) can replace a 3-ounce serving of meat, poultry, or fish.

Eggs

No more than 3 to 4 egg yolks per week.

Use an egg white plus 2 teaspoons of unsaturated oil to replace a whole egg when cooking. Cholesterol-free commercial egg substitutes are also good.

Vegetables and fruits

5 or more servings a day; serving size is 1 medium piece of fruit or ½ cup fruit juice; ½–1 cup cooked or raw vegetables.

Choose from: all vegetables and fruits except coconut. Olives and avocados should be counted as fats. Starchy vegetables (potatoes, corn, lima beans, yams) count as pasta and bread selections.

Milk products

2 or more servings per day over 24 years old; serving size is 1 cup skim or low-fat milk; 1 cup nonfat or low-fat yogurt; 1 oz. low-fat cheese or ½ cup low-fat cottage cheese.

Choose from: milk products with 1–2% fat; buttermilk made from skim or 1% fat; nonfat or low-fat yogurt; low-fat cheeses.

Breads, cereals, pasta, and starchy vegetables

6 or more servings per day; serving size: 1 slice bread, ¼ cup nugget type cereal; ½ cup hot cereal; 1 cup cooked rice or pasta; ¼–½ cup starchy vegetables; 1 cup low-fat soup.

Choose from: wheat, rye, raisin breads; water (not egg) bagels; crackers (graham, rye, oyster, saltine); air-popped popcorn; rice and pasta, potatoes, corn, lima beans, green peas.

Fats and oils

No more than 5–8 servings per day. Serving size: 1 teaspoon vegetable oil or regular margarine; 2 teaspoons diet margarine; 1 tablespoon salad dressing; 2 teaspoons mayonnaise or peanut butter; 3 teaspoons seeds or nuts; ⅛ medium avocado; 10 small or 5 large olives.

Choose from: vegetable oils such as canola, corn, olive, safflower, sesame, soybean, sunflower.

Appendix C-2: Eating to Reduce Cancer Risk

The U.S. Department of Health and Human Services, the U.S. Department of Agriculture, and the National Academy of Sciences all recommend that you eat a balanced diet low in fat and which includes at least 5 servings a day of fruits and vegetables. Because they are low in fat, high in fiber, and contain vitamins A and C, fruits and vegetables can help reduce your risk of cancer. They also help promote a healthy digestive tract.

Eat a variety of fruits and vegetables every day, but especially those high in fiber and in vitamins A and C. Include several servings a week from the family of vegetables called cruciferous (related to the cabbage family), such as broccoli and cauliflower.

∽   ∽   ∽

Tips for Eating 5 Fruit and Vegetable Servings a Day

Morning Drink a glass of juice.
Add sliced bananas or strawberries to your cereal.
Have a bowl of fruit, such as melon or peaches.
Top your pancakes with fruit instead of syrup.

Lunch Have a salad or soup that contains vegetables.
Add zucchini, carrot, or celery sticks to your brown bag lunch.
Eat a piece of fruit like an apple or an orange, or a couple of plums or kiwis.
Add lettuce, sprouts, or tomatoes to your sandwich.

Snack Nibble on some grapes or raisins.
Take along some dried fruit like apricots, prunes, or figs.
Choose a glass of juice.
Keep cut raw vegetables in water in the refrigerator.

Dinner Add vegetables to your main dish such as broccoli to a pasta entrée or casserole.

Add raw vegetables or fruit to your green salad.
Use fruits as a garnish on main dishes.
Order extra vegetables when you are eating out.

Dessert   Liven up a plain dessert with fresh fruit.
Top frozen yogurt with pineapple or papaya.
Add chopped fruit or berries to muffins, cakes, or
cookies.

Source: "Eat More Fruits and Vegetables—5 a Day for Better Health," U.S. Department of Health and Human Services, Public Health Services, National Institutes of Health; NIH Publication No. 92-3248; October 1991.

Height and Weight Table

Please note: This table is for reference purposes, and should not always be used literally. You may want to discuss these weight ranges with your physician. Take into consideration how you feel at your present weight, keeping in mind the principles from Chapter 2 about not distorting your own reality to an unattainable ideal.

Suggested Weights for Adults—USDA

Height	35 Years or Older
5' 0"	108–138
5' 1"	111–143
5' 2"	115–148
5' 3"	119–152
5' 4"	122–157
5' 5"	126–162
5' 6"	130–167
5' 7"	134–172
5' 8"	138–178
5' 9"	142–183
5' 10"	146–188

Note: Height is in stocking feet and weight is without clothes.
The USDA does not distinguish in this table between men and women.

The ranges here are much more liberal than the Metropolitan Life Insurance tables, which were updated in 1983 from the more stringent 1959 ranges. (For example, the range for a medium frame 5'6" woman was 124–139; in 1983 the same size woman's range was listed as 130–144.)

GLOSSARY

Abstract A summary or abridgment of an article, book, or research study.

Acupressure Massage in which pressure is applied to the body at the same locations that would be used for acupuncture. See *shiatsu*.

Acupuncture Chinese therapeutic practice of inserting thin needles into specific points on the body.

Adaptogenic herbs According to Eastern and alternative practitioners, herbs that stimulate the body's immune system to encourage self-regulation.

Amenorrhea Absence or abnormal cessation of menstruation.

Androgen Male hormone.

Anecdotal Based on descriptions of unmatched individual cases rather than on controlled, statistical studies.

Anovulatory cycles Menstrual cycles when no egg is released from the ovaries.

Arthralgia Joint pain.

Atresia Degeneration.

Atrophic urethritis Inflammation of the urethra due to tissue thinning; a condition that can be caused by estrogen depletion.

Autoclave sterilized Sterilized in a device using superheated steam under pressure.

Beta-adrenergic blockers Drugs used to manage high blood pressure.

Biofeedback Technique that enables a person to increase alpha brain wave activity to achieve a state of relaxation.

Bok choy Chinese cabbage.

Bone density study   A measurement of bone mineral content and density to determine skeletal health. Various methods are used.

Bone remodeling   A process that takes place continuously inside the bone marrow, where large multinuclear cells (osteoblasts) act on old bone cells and break them down (a process called resorption). Then new bone is formed, and the cycle repeats.

Breakthrough bleeding   Vaginal bleeding between regular menstrual periods.

Breast biopsy   Removal and microscopic examination of tumor tissue to confirm or rule out breast cancer; performed on an outpatient basis under local anesthetic.

Breast self-examination (BSE)   A technique that enables a woman to detect palpable (able to be felt) changes in her breasts, useful as an adjunct to regular mammography screening in the early detection of breast cancer. BSE should be done once a month soon after the completion of the menstrual period and on a monthly basis after menopause.

Calcitonin (salmon-calcitonin)   Pharmaceutical alternative to hormones for preventing loss of bone calcium.

Calcitriol   An injectable form of vitamin D that promotes calcium absorption.

Calcium citrate   A form of calcium that is more readily absorbed; sometimes recommended as a supplement for women over 60.

Catecholamines   Biologically active amines, epinephrine and norepinephrine, derived from the amino acid tyrosine. They have a marked effect on the nervous and cardiovascular systems, metabolic rate, temperature, and smooth muscle.

Cervical canal   Passageway between the vagina and the uterus.

Cervix   The lower, narrow end of the uterus; the "neck" of the uterus.

Cholelithiasis   Presence of gallstones.

Climacteric   The period from perimenopause to cessation of menopausal symptoms. From the Greek *klimakter,* "a rung of the ladder."

Conjugated estrogens   Combined estrogens from the urine of pregnant mares. Contained in one of the most widely prescribed oral estrogens, Premarin.

Corpus luteum   A yellowish mass or casing that forms where the egg was released and secretes progesterone. See *luteinizing hormone.*

Cruciferous   Family of plants including cabbage, broccoli, and mustard greens, thought to be useful as cancer preventives.

Diastolic pressure   In blood pressure readings, the lower number, which measures the pressure between beats. See *systolic pressure.*

Diethylstilbestrol (DES)   A synthetic preparation possessing estrogenic properties. Its use during pregnancy has been found to be related to subsequent malignancies of the reproductive system in the daughters of mothers who were so treated.

Dilation and curettage (D&C)   A scraping of the uterine wall.

Dong quai   An adaptogenic herb that contains phytoestrogens (plant estrogens) used in the Orient to treat hot flashes, anxiety, depression, and insomnia. See *adaptogenic herbs.*

Double-blind study   A study in which neither researchers nor participants know which volunteers are taking the drug being studied and which are taking the placebo. See *placebo.*

Dowager's hump   Hunched back; a symptom of osteoporosis.

Dual energy X-ray absorptiometry (DEXA)   Sophisticated, noninvasive laser scanning X ray of the hip and lumbar spine to measure bone density.

Dysfunctional bleeding   Unpredictable or unusually heavy uterine bleeding.

Dyspareunia   Difficult or painful intercourse.

Dysphoric mood   State of unhappiness.

Embolism   Sudden blocking of an artery by a clot.

Endogenous estrogen   Estrogen originating within the body.

Endometrial biopsy   Excision of a small piece of uterine tissue for microscopic examination.

Endometrium   Lining of the uterus.

Endorphins Natural opiates with pain-relieving properties produced by the body.

Epidemiologists Scientists who study factors that cause and influence the incidence and distribution of disease in entire populations.

Estradiol The most potent of three estrogen compounds made in the body. Produced by the ovary, it is part of the complicated feedback system between the hypothalamus, pituitary gland, and ovary that results in the normal monthly ovulatory cycle.

Estriol A relatively weak estrogen compound, produced as a by-product of estradiol and estrone metabolism.

Estrogen Female sex hormones naturally produced in the ovaries and responsible for development of reproductive organs and female secondary sex characteristics. Natural estrogen production is increased during ovulation, pregnancy, and menstruation. Exogenous estrogens (see below) are used in oral contraceptives and to relieve menopausal symptoms.

Estrogen receptor-positive Able to bind with and be affected by estrogen.

Estrone A low-level estrogen compound converted from androgens in fatty tissue.

Estropipate A synthetic estrogen.

Estrus cycle Recurring changes in the reproductive organs caused by ovarian hormonal activity.

Etiology Study of causes or origins of disease.

Exogenous estrogen Estrogen that has been developed outside the body, either synthetically or biologically.

Fallopian tube One of two passageways through which an ovum travels from an ovary to the uterus.

Fibrocystic disease A benign condition of the breasts in which clumps of tissue occasionally produce noncancerous lumps.

Fluoride Chemical compound that incorporates into the structure of bone and teeth and may improve bone density; still under study as a treatment for osteoporosis.

Follicle stimulating hormone (FSH) A hormone secreted by the pituitary that stimulates the ovaries.

FSH blood tests Tests to determine presence of follicle stimulating hormones; a high level of FSH indicates diminished ovarian function and menopause.

Generativity Concern with and motivation to contribute something to future generations.

Ginseng A Chinese herb (root). One use is as an alternative treatment for menopausal symptoms (hot flashes, insomnia, agitated depression, regulating blood sugar, or premenopausal exhaustion).

Gonadotropins Hormones that stimulate the ovaries, such as FSH or LH. See *follicle stimulating hormone* and *luteinizing hormone.*

Graafian follicle A mature vesicular follicle of the ovary. Beginning with puberty and continuing until menopause, except during pregnancy, a graafian follicle develops at approximately monthly intervals. Each follicle contains a nearly mature ovum, which is discharged from the ovary upon rupture of the follicle, a process called ovulation. See *ovulation.*

High-density lipoprotein (HDL) The "good" cholesterol.

Homeopathy System of medical practice that treats disease by giving small doses of remedies; in healthy persons, the remedies would produce mild symptoms of the disease treated.

Hormone replacement therapy (HRT) A regimen of hormones in combination, most usually estrogen and synthetic progestin, prescribed short term for treatment of uncomfortable menopausal symptoms and long term for prevention of osteoporosis and cardiovascular disease.

Hot flash Also called hot flush. A sudden sweating and reddening of the skin, especially face and torso, its cause unknown. Sometimes preceded by an "aura."

Hypercholesterolemia Excessive amount of cholesterol in the blood; usually a hereditary condition.

Hyperplasia An abnormal growth of cells, an indication of a possible precancerous condition.

Hyperthyroidism A condition caused by excessive secretion of the thyroid glands, which increases the basal metabolic rate, causing an increased demand for food to support this metabolic activity.

Hypoestrogenic Having a diminished amount of estrogen in the blood, as in menopause.

Hypothalamus An area of the brain located above the pituitary gland; controls many involuntary bodily functions and regulates the pituitary gland.

Hysterectomy Surgical removal of the uterus.

Interiority The turning inward of thoughts and increased contemplation in old age.

Intraductal carcinoma in situ Cancer growth that has not spread and is contained within a duct (e.g., a breast duct); the most curable of all breast cancers.

Kegel exercises Exercises for strengthening the perineal muscles of the female; can help to prevent incontinence.

Labia Folds of skin on either side of the vulva and the opening of the vagina.

Libido Sexual desire.

Low-density lipoprotein (LDL) The "bad" cholesterol. See *high-density lipoprotein.*

Luteinizing hormone (LH) Hormone secreted by the anterior lobe of the pituitary that stimulates development of the corpus luteum. See *corpus luteum.*

Menarche The onset of menses.

Menopause The period that marks the permanent cessation of menstrual activity.

Meridians Longitudinal lines or pathways on the body where acupuncture points are located.

Mexican yam A plant that contains small amounts of natural progesterone; sometimes recommended by alternative practitioners for symptoms of menopause.

Myalgia Generalized muscle pain.

Naturopath One who practices a therapeutic system that does not use drugs or therapy but employs natural forces such as light, heat, air, water, and massage.

Noncontraceptive estrogen Exogenous estrogen in HRT used to relieve menopausal symptoms, in contrast to estrogen used in oral contraceptives. See *hormone replacement therapy.*

Nonhormonal Referring to a treatment for menopause that does not involve hormones or HRT.

Noninvasive Not penetrating the skin (as by surgery or hypodermic needle or endoscope).

Nulliparous Never having borne a child.

Oophorectomy Removal of the ovaries only.

Opiates Naturally occurring brain chemicals that produce effects similar to those of the drug opium. See *endorphins.*

Osteoblasts Large multinuclear cells in the bone marrow.

Osteopenia Loss of bone mass.

Osteoporosis The "brittle bones" disease; an increased porosity of the bones.

Ovulation The periodic ripening and rupture of the mature graafian follicle and the discharge of the ovum from the cortex of the ovary. Ovulation occurs approximately 14 days before the start of the next menstrual period. See *graafian follicle.*

Perimenopause The time around, or just prior to, menopause.

Phytogens Plant estrogens.

Pituitary A small gland at the base of the brain that secretes hormones controlling growth and reproduction.

Placebo Inactive substance used in controlled studies of drugs. The placebo is given to a group of participants (the control group) and the drug being tested is given to a similar group; then the results obtained in the two groups are compared. See *double-blind study.*

Postmenopausal After the menopause transition period and menstrual cycles have stopped, usually for a period of six months to one year.

Premature menopause   A natural menopause that comes before age 40.

Premenopausal   Before menopause (average age of menopause is 50).

Primiparity   The first full-term pregnancy.

Progestin   Synthetic progesterone prescribed for use alone or in combination with estrogen.

Prophylactic   A preventive measure.

Psychogenic   Referring to a symptom caused by mental factors rather than organic factors.

Pulmonary embolism   Closure of the pulmonary artery or one of its branches by a blood clot.

Rapid eye movement (REM)   Cyclic movement of the closed eyes during sleep. Often referred to as "deep sleep," this period of sleep is strongly associated with dreaming.

Reflexology   Massage involving finger pressure, especially to the feet.

Remodeling   In the bone, the process of breaking down and renewal of bone tissue. See *bone remodeling*.

Reproductive endocrinology   A subspecialty in the field of gynecology that requires additional training and board certification in the endocrinology of the reproductive system.

Resorption   The dissolution and assimilation of tissue.

Sexual dysfunction   Impaired sexual activity or function caused by mental or organic factors.

Shiatsu   Type of massage in which pressure is applied to the same areas of the body as those targeted in acupuncture. See *acupressure*.

Steroids (anabolic)   Testosterone-like synthetic hormones used to promote muscle growth and repair of body tissues. Anabolic steroid use can have short-term and long-term harmful effects, one of them being thinner bones.

Stress fracture   Bone fracture caused by repeated application of a heavy load (such as the constant pounding on a surface by runners); osteoporosis increases incidence of stress fractures.

Stress incontinence   Inability to prevent escape of urine during stress such as laughing, coughing, or sneezing. A common consequence of vaginal delivery and aging.

Surgical menopause   Condition of estrogen depletion caused by a complete hysterectomy (removal of the uterus and ovaries) or removal of the ovaries only.

Systolic pressure   In blood pressure readings, the upper number, which measures the pressure of blood flow from the heart. See *diastolic pressure.*

Thrombophlebitis   Blood clots in a vein.

Tofu   A protein-rich food made of soybean curd.

Transdermal   Method of delivering medication by absorption through the skin without injection.

Unopposed estrogens   Oral or injectable estrogen without the addition of progesterone.

Urogenital   Involving both the urinary and genital structures or functions.

Uterine leiomyoma   Fibroids; benign tumors of the uterus.

Vaginal atrophy   A dryness and thinning of the vaginal wall.

Vaginal mucosa   Lubricating mucous membrane of the vagina.

Vaginismus   Involuntary, painful muscle spasms of the vagina.

Vaginitis   Inflammation of the vagina.

Venous thrombosis   Presence of blood clots impeding blood flow in the veins; most often occurring in the legs or pelvis.

Weight-bearing exercise   Exercise in which a load is placed on the skeleton, through a high- or low-impact aerobics routine, walking, or lifting weights.

BIBLIOGRAPHY

American Cancer Society. *Selected Cancers, Facts and Figures* 1999, www.cancer.org.

American Cancer Society. "Surveillance Research, 1995." *Breast Cancer Facts and Figures,* 1996.

American College of Obstetricians and Gynecologists. "Hormone Replacement Therapy." *ACOG Educational Bulletin,* no. 247 (May 1998): 1–8.

Bachmann, Gloria A., M.D. "The Changes Before 'The Change.'" *Postgraduate Medicine* 95, no. 4 (March 1994): 117–22.

Brownlee, Shannon. "The Menopause Myth." *Working Woman* 18, no. 12 (December 1993): 80–84.

Butler, Kurt. *A Consumer's Guide to Alternative Medicine.* Buffalo, NY: Prometheus Books, 1992.

CRISP (Computer Retrieval of Information on Scientific Projects), commons.cit.nih.gov/crisp/owa.cris.

Cutler, Winnifred B., Ph.D., and Celso-Ramon Garcia, M.D. *Menopause: A Guide for Women and Those Who Love Them,* revised ed. New York: W. W. Norton & Co., 1993.

Eastman, Peggy. "ACS Vigorously Defends Mammography Screening for Women in Their 40s." *Oncology Times* 16, no. 1 (January 1994): 28–29.

Fuchs, Nan Kathryn, Ph.D. "Yogurt, Cheese and Milk: Good Fast Food?" *Women's Health Letter* (March 1994): 1–2.

Fugh-Berman, Adriane. "Estriol: A Kinder, Gentler Estrogen?" *Alternative Therapies in Women's Health* 12, no. 6 (June 1999): 52–53.

Gaby, Alan R., M.D. *Preventing and Reversing Osteoporosis.* Rocklin, CA: Prima Publishing, 1994.

Gambrell, R. Don, Jr., M.D. *Estrogen Replacement Therapy User Guide*. Dallas: Essential Medical Information Systems, 1989.

Gaudoin, Tina. "The Return of the Real Woman." *Mirabella* (April 1994): 42–46.

Greendale, Gail A., M.D., and Howard L. Judd, M.D. "The Menopause: Health Implications and Clinical Management." *Journal of the American Geriatrics Society* 41, no. 4 (April 1993): 426–36.

Greer, Germaine. *The Change: Women, Aging and the Menopause*. New York: Fawcett Columbine, 1993.

Gutfeld, Greg, et al. "Relax the Flash." *Prevention* 45, no. 3 (March 1993): 18–19.

Henkel, Gretchen. "Quality of Medical Information on Internet Varies, Study Finds." *Oncology Times*, no. 9 (1999): 33–35.

———. "The Status of Oncology Research in Complementary and Alternative Medicine: Attitudes Changing in Government and Practice Levels." *Oncology Times*, no. 5 (1999): 55–60.

———. "Wanted: Alternative Treatments for Menopause in Breast Cancer Survivors." *Oncology Times* 15, no. 1 (January 1993): 8–10.

"History of Women's Health Initiative," www.nhlbi.nih.gov/index.htm.

"Hormones Reconsidered as Best Treatment." *San Luis Obispo County Tribune*, May 1, 1999, 3.

Hulley, et al. "Randomized Trial of Estrogen Plus Progestin for Secondary Prevention of Coronary Heart Disease in Postmenopausal Women. Heart and Estrogen/Progestin Replacement Study (HERS) Research Group." *Journal of the American Medical Association*, no. 7 (August 19, 1998): 605–13.

Kaplan, Carolyn, M.D., associate clinical professor, Emory University School of Medicine, Atlanta, Georgia, interview with author, July 8, 1999.

Lindsay, Robert, M.D., Ph.D., chief of internal medicine, Helen Hayes Regional Bone Center, West Haverstraw, New York, interview with author, May 10, 1999.

Lindheim, Steven R., M.D., and Morris Notelovitz, M.D., "The Independent Effects of Exercise and Estrogen on Lipids and Lipoproteins in Postmenopausal Women." *Obstetrics and Gynecology* (February 1994, 1983): 167–72.

Lott, Deborah, Gretchen Henkel, and Marvin Karno, M.D. "How to Choose a Psychotherapist." *UCLA Health Insights* (December 1985): 3–4.

Love, Susan M., M.D., with Karen Lindsey. *Dr. Susan Love's Breast Book.* Reading, MA: Addison-Wesley Publishing Co., 1991.

"Low Dose HRT Prevents Bone Loss," *Doctors Guide*, www.pslgroup.com.

Murdaugh, Carolyn L., R.N., Ph.D. "Gender Differences in Heart Disease," paper presented at 61st Annual Fall Symposium, American Heart Association, Los Angeles, September 8, 1993.

Nachtigall, Lila E., M.D., and Joan Rattner Heilman. *Estrogen: The Facts Can Change Your Life!* New York: Harper Perennial, 1991.

Notelovitz, Morris, M.D., Ph.D., and Diana Tonnessen. *Menopause and Midlife Health.* New York: St. Martin's Press, 1994.

Ochs, Ridgely. "That Spare Tire Can Mean Trouble." *Los Angeles Times,* October 4, 1992, B-3.

"Patient Info, Medications and Osteoporosis," National Osteoporosis Foundation, www.nof.org.

Pinn, Vivian W., M.D. "Commentary: Women, Research, and the National Institutes of Health." *American Journal of Preventive Medicine* 8, no. 5 (1992): 324–27.

"Progestins and Progesterone." *A Friend Indeed* XI, no. 1 (January 1998): 1–8, www.afriendindeed.ca.

Randall, Teri. "Women Need More and Better Information on Menopause from Their Physicians, Says Survey." *Journal of the American Medical Association* 270, no. 14 (October 13, 1993): 1664.

Renner, John , M.D. Kansas City, Missouri, interview with author, January 7, 1994.

Sachs, Judith. *What Women Should Know About Menopause*. New York: Dell Medical Library, 1991.

Sarrel, Philip M., M.D. "Psychosexual Effects of Menopause: Role of Androgens." *American Journal of Obstetrics and Gynecology* 180, no. 3, part 2 (March 1999): 319–24.

———. "Sexuality in the Middle Years." *Obstetrics and Gynecology Clinics of North America* 14, no. 1 (March 1987): 50–62.

Sheehy, Gail. *Menopause: The Silent Passage*. New York: Random House, 1998.

Shumaker, S. A., et al. "The Women's Health Initiative Memory Study (WHIMS): A Trial of the Effect of Estrogen Therapy in Preventing and Slowing the Progression of Dementia." *Controlled Clinical Trials* 19, no. 6 (December 1998): 604–21.

Skelly, Flora Johnson. "Millions in Menopause." *American Medical News* (July 27, 1992): 28–31.

Speroff, Leon, M.D., Robert H. Glass, M.D., and Nathan Kase, M.D. *Clinical Gynecologic Endocrinology and Infertility*, 4th ed. Baltimore: Williams & Wilkins, 1989.

Stevens-Long, Judith. *Adult Life*, 3d ed. Mountain View, CA: Mayfield Publishing Co., 1988.

Stumpf, Paul G., M.D., clinical professor of obstetrics, gynecology, and reproductive sciences, Robert Wood Johnson Medical School, New Brunswick, New Jersey, interview with author, May 13, 1999. *Taber's Cyclopedic Medical Dictionary*, 14th ed. Philadelphia: F. A. Davis Co., 1981.

Utian, Wulf H., M.D., Ph.D., and Ruth Jacobowitz. *Managing Your Menopause*. New York: Simon and Schuster, 1990.

Weinberger, et al., "Long-Term Efficacy of Nonsurgical Urinary Incontinence Treatment in Elderly Women." *Journal of Gerontology and Biological Science and Medical Science* 54, no. 3 (March 1999): 117–21.

Zisla, Bonita D., M.F.C.C., and Susan Swadener, Ph.D., R.D., interview with author, May 14, 1999.

INDEX